I0493851

Published by ENDOCRINE EDUCATION,INC and MDTEXT.COM,INC, South Dartmouth, MA
1 June 2014. All rights reserved.

ISBN-13: 978-1499618716

ISBN-10: 1499618719

A SPECIAL SYMPOSIUM Presented by
WWW.ENDOTEXT.ORG and WWW.THYROIDMANAGER.ORG

TYROSINE KINASE INHIBITORS
IN MANAGEMENT OF AGGRESSIVE
DIFFERENTIATED THYROID CANCER

Organized and Edited by James V Hennessey, MD and Leslie J De Groot,MD

INTRODUCTION

James V Hennessey, MD, FACP
Division of Endocrinology, Beth Israel Deaconess Medical Center, Boston, MA

S1- CONTEMPORARY MANAGEMENT OF DIFFERENTIATED THYROID CANCER

Furio Pacini, MD Thyroid Unit, University of Siena, Siena Italy
Leslie J De Groot, MD, University of Rhode Island, Providence, RI

S2- DEFINING RAI REFRACTORY THYROID CANCER: WHEN IS RAI THERAPY UNLIKELY TO ACHIEVE A THERAPEUTIC RESPONSE?

R Michael Tuttle, MD and Mona M. Sabra, MD
Endocrinology Service, Memorial Sloan-Kettering Cancer Center, New York, New York, 10021

S3- SELECTION OF PATIENTS FOR TYROSINE KINASE INHIBITOR TREATMENT

Martin Schlumberger , MD Professor of Oncology, University of Paris-Sud, Director, Nuclear Medicine and Endocrine Tumors Division, Institut Gustave-Roussy, Villejuif, Paris, France.
Furio Pacini, MD Professor of Endocrinology, Director, Section of Endocrinology and Metabolism, University of Siena, Siena, Italy

S4- NEW TREATMENT ALGORITHMS FOR SYSTEMIC THERAPY WITH TKIs IN MANAGING AGGRESSIVE THYROID CANCER

Joshua Klopper, MD and Bryan Haugen, MD
University of Colorado School of Medicine

S5--FUTURE DIRECTIONS IN THERAPY OF ADVANCED THYROID CANCER.

James A. Fagin, MD[1] and Alan Ho, MD[2]
Human Oncology and Pathogenesis Program[1] and Department of Medicine[2], Memorial Sloan-Kettering Cancer Center, New York, NY.

INTRODUCTION

The contemporary treatment of thyroid cancer has evolved greatly in the past 30 years. This advancement in knowledge has been more rapid than in the preceding century and continues to be a challenge to the practicing endocrinologist. This symposium on advances in the diagnosis and treatment of thyroid cancer was developed to summarize the current state of the art in identification and management of the majority of thyroid cancers encountered while alerting the clinician to the characteristics of more advanced cases which have a far less favorable outcomes.

The first chapter of this work focuses on the current management of differentiated thyroid cancer. An outline of the diagnostic tools commonly implemented in the assessment of patients sets the stage for a discussion of the clinical course of the most common types of differentiated thyroid cancer, culminating with an extensive review of therapeutic interventions. After selecting an appropriate initial surgical procedure, it is evident that further clinical decisions are based on the stage of disease present post operatively. The need for further interventions such as 131-I ablation and TSH suppressive therapy with l-thyroxine are determined by the extent of initial surgery, the risk predicted by the histopathologic findings and the predicted effectiveness of these interventions. Follow up strategies using available clinical laboratory and imaging techniques are laid out in detail. Restaging and further treatments based on clinical findings are detailed as are considerations for the safe administration of therapeutic interventions and the potential for side effects of the same. Long term surveillance strategies and prognoses are made clear as well as suggestions for optimal outcomes are made clear.

The second section of this work introduces the concept of 131-I refractory (more advanced) differentiated thyroid cancer. After a brief review of the clinical history of 131-I therapy in patients with differentiated thyroid cancer, Tuttle and Sabra review factors which are associated with suboptimal 131-I avidity in metastatic thyroid cancer and explain methods of assessing the potential for successful use of 131-I to treat patients with more advanced thyroid cancer. A thorough explanation of several methods of dosimetry are outlined including the advantages and limitations of each in predicating the effectiveness of 131-I in improving patient outcomes. This section is summarized with a set of practical findings to guide clinical decision making and defining 131-I refractory disease where further use of 131-I would not likely result in improved patient outcomes and may only be expected to be associated with the toxicities of radioactive iodine.

The selection of patients with advanced thyroid cancer for more advanced intervention with tyrosine kinase inhibitor (TKI) therapies is the focus of the next section of this symposium. Pacini and Schlumberger re-define the limited life expectancy predicted for those with more advanced thyroid cancer as defined as 131-I refractory metastatic disease. These authors review the methods employed to assess the extent and course of the minority of differentiated thyroid cancer who have persistent of recurrent metastatic disease despite the apparently highly effective conventional treatments outlined by Pacini and DeGroot in the first chapter. This section proposes principles of clinical management of such individuals which range from continued TSH suppressive therapy with LT4 and active surveillance, appropriate in some with non-progressive disease, to revisional surgery for symptomatic focal disease or the institution of advanced TKI interventions when progression of the thyroid cancer is clear. An introduction to TKI selection closes out this section and sets the stage for the next discussion.

Klopper and Haugen have provided us with an overview of the current state of modern systemic therapies for managing aggressive thyroid cancer when traditional interventions are no longer effective. These authors define the mechanisms of action of the of the multi-targeted tyrosine kinase inhibitors. They provide us with an overview of the current state of knowledge of TKI therapies in thyroid cancer trials with especial attribution of the targets of each of the agents utilized. Trial outcomes are detailed so as to provide a useful overview of potentially useful interventions for these unfortunate patients with advancing disease. The authors summarize the current impact that these agents have had on clinical practice and propose an algorithm for assessing candidates for advanced systemic therapy of thyroid cancer and propose a very practical construct to support the ongoing administration of these therapies with periodic re-staging and appropriate monitoring in the short and long term.

Finally, Fagin and HO have provided us with a comprehensive discussion of experience with multi-kinase inhibitors emphasizing the positives and limitations of these therapies in the current literature. They briefly discuss a limited role for cytotoxic chemotherapeutic agents especially for anaplastic thyroid cancer cases where traditional surgical and 131-I interventions are of limited value and point out that TKIs also have been demonstrated to have limited utility. The remainder of this elegant view forward is dedicated to explaining efforts to target the genetic drivers of thyroid cancer, enhance the effectiveness of 131-I in those grown refractory and overcome adaptive resistance to some small molecule inhibitors in some advanced thyroid cancers. Finally the authors explore the future of cancer immunotherapies in advanced thyroid cancer patients over all leaving us with a clear understanding of current directions in developing ever more advanced treatments for the patient presenting the dilemma of recurrent, 131-I resistant and advancing metastatic thyroid cancer.

James V Hennessey M D FACP
Director, Clinical Endocrinology
Division of Endocrinology
Beth Israel Deaconess Medical Center

S1-CONTEMPORARY MANAGEMENT OF DIFFERENTIATED THYROID CANCER

Furio Pacini, MD Thyroid Unit, University of Siena, Siena Italy
Leslie J De Groot, MD, University of Rhode Island, Providence, RI

Some of the material in this chapter has appeared in other discussions of Thyroid cancer treatment (in www.thyroidmanager.org) and is used here with permission from Endocrine Education, Inc.

DIAGNOSIS
Management of differentiated thyroid cancer begins with diagnosis, usually surgical excision, and initial staging postoperatively. Diagnosis is achieved by history and exam, thyroid function tests and calcitonin (CT) assay, ultrasound, most frequently fine needle aspiration (FNA), sometimes isotope scans radiographs, computed axial tomography (CAT) scans or magnetic resonance imaging (MRI), and even positron emission tomography (PET) scans. Diagnostic methods and concepts are extensively reviewed in www.thyroidmanager.org/thyroidcancer to which readers are referred.
Thyrotropin (TSH), free thyroxine (fT4) and thyroid peroxidase antibody (TPO-Ab) assays are needed to document the patient's metabolic status and fitness for operation, to rule out a possible hyper functioning thyroid lesion, and sometimes to help differentiate thyroiditis as the etiology of the lesion of interest. Serum TG measurement is not recommended in routine practice preoperatively because elevated levels are associated with any thyroid growth. Ultrasound exam is currently central to diagnosis, providing information on the size, shape and number of lesions, probability of infiltrative disease, and of involved neck nodes. The key test is of course FNA and its interpretation, supplemented sometimes by assay of tumor genetic markers that can augment, or reduce, the statistical probability that the tumor is malignant. Whole body (WB) Scans for diagnosis of metastatic disease are performed if there is some suggestion of disease spread, but are more commonly conducted after operation. The results of the diagnostic workup may include definite or possible thyroid cancer within a nodule or thyroid lobe, and possible nodal or metastatic disease. Management of cancer in children, and of anaplastic and medullary tumors, is reviewed in Thyroidmanager.

COURSE OF DISEASE
Management should be guided by an understanding of the natural history of papillary and follicular thyroid cancers. Age at diagnosis has an important bearing on the patient's subsequent course. The adverse effect of age on prognosis increases gradually with each decade (1). For practical assessment purposes, it is clear that patients diagnosed before age 45 have a much better prognosis than those detected later (2). Age is also directly related to the incidence of undifferentiated tumors and to overall mortality. Pregnancy does not seem to worsen the course of established or previously treated

thyroid cancer (3). Overall, women have a better prognosis than men with thyroid cancer (4). Other characteristics of the tumor, including (as would be expected) distant metastases, extra-glandular extension, gross invasion of the tumor capsule, and increasing size also carry a worsened prognosis (4).

Papillary carcinoma has a peak incidence in the third and fourth decades (5). It occurs three times more frequently in women than in men, and accounts for 60-70% of all thyroid cancers in adults and about 70% of those found in children. The disease tends to remain localized in the thyroid gland and in time metastasizes locally to the cervical or upper mediastinal nodes. The lesions are multicentric in 20% or more of patients, especially in children. Using rigid pathologic criteria, perhaps two-thirds of predominantly papillary thyroid cancers are found to have follicular elements. The natural history of these tumors is generally considered similar to that of pure papillary lesions (6). Metastases may conform to either histologic pattern. At present, the mixed tumors are lumped together with all other papillary cancers. This tumor tends to be indolent and may exist for decades without killing the host. In a Mayo Clinic series of papillary tumors that were detected because of lymph node metastasis or found incidentally during surgery of the thyroid gland, all the patients were unaffected by the tumors over several decades (5). The presentation of papillary thyroid cancer has been changing in the last two decades compared to previous years, with an increasing number of small tumors and less frequent lymph node metastases at presentation (7)

Many papillary tumors present as occult or "minimal' cancers, incidentally found at neck ultrasound, and measure under 0.5-1 cm in size. The term occult has been used in a variety of ways, including reference to tumors with malignant lymph nodes but no obvious primary, or in reference to tumors under 1.5 cm in diameter. Currently the preferred term is microcarcinoma. Mayo Clinic reports of papillary tumors under 1.5 cm in diameter, treated with conservative subtotal thyroidectomy and node dissection, have stressed their non-lethal nature, but a 1980 follow-up report on 820 patients treated by this group notes that 6 (0.7%) patients eventually died after spread of tumor from such "occult" primaries (8). Patients with appropriately treated minimal tumors have 96-100% survival after 15-30 years.

While the disease may be aggressive in children, it is distinctly less aggressive in young adults, as compared to patients over age 40 (4).Young patients tend to have small primary lesions and extensive adenopathy, but even with local invasion survival is good (9). When papillary cancer occurs in persons over the age of 45, it may show, on microscopic examination, areas of undifferentiation, and pursue a more highly malignant clinical course. The lesions tend to be larger and more infiltrative, and to have fewer local metastases (10). It is possible that persons apparently dying of thyroid cancer in older age actually have had their disease for many years, and that it has simply evolved into a more malignant phase (11, 12).

Papillary carcinoma tends to metastasize locally to lymph nodes, and occasionally produces cystic structures near the thyroid that are difficult to diagnose because of the paucity of malignant tissue. In this case measurement of thyroglobulin in the fluid aspirate is a clue for the correct diagnosis. The presence of nodal metastasis correlates with recurrence but has little effect on mortality in patients under age 45. In patients over 45, the presence of nodes is associated with greater recurrence rates and more deaths (14, 15).

The tumors often metastasize elsewhere, especially to lung or bones. Papillary tumors may metastasize to the lungs and produce a few nodules, or the lung fields may have a snowflake appearance throughout. These tumors are amazingly well tolerated and may allow relatively normal physical activity for 10-30 years. At times, particularly in the follicular variant of papillary thyroid cancer, the pulmonary metastases are active in forming thyroid hormone, and may even function as a source of hormone supply after thyroidectomy. The metastases may progress gradually and result in obstructive and restrictive pulmonary disease. They also may develop arteriovenous shunts, with hypoxia or cyanosis. Such shunts become more prominent during pregnancy, perhaps as an effect of the increased supply of estrogens. The tall cell variant of papillary carcinoma comprises about 10% of total cases, and as noted by several authors appears to be more aggressive than other forms of the disease (16.17). .

The usual net extra mortality in papillary cancer is not great when compared to that of a control population, perhaps 10-20% over 20-30 years (12, 13, and 15). Mortality is rare in patients diagnosed before age 40, and is mainly observed in patients found to have invasive or metastatic disease at initial diagnosis. About one-half of patients ultimately dying from this lesion do so because of local invasion.
We found that risk of death from cancer was increased by extrathyroidal invasion (6 fold) or distant metastasis (47 fold), age over 45 years (32 fold) and size over 3 cm (6 fold). Thyroiditis, multifocality and the presence of neck nodes had no effect on disease-induced mortality.

Follicular carcinoma has a peak incidence in the fifth decade of life in the United States and accounts for about one-quarter of all thyroid carcinomas (4, 18, and 19). It is often a slowly growing tumor and frequently is recognized as a nodule in the thyroid gland before metastases appear. Variation in the cellular pattern ranges from an almost normal-appearing structure to anaplastic tissue that forms no follicles or colloid. The insular variant of follicular thyroid cancer tends to be more aggressive (20). The tumor is three times as common in women as in men. At operation one-half to two-thirds of these tumors are resectable. Tumors that are small and well circumscribed (not surprisingly) tend to be less lethal than those actively infiltrating local structures at the initial operation. Local adenopathy, which is uncommon, probably carries a greater risk, and extensive invasion of the tumor capsule and thyroid tissue increases mortality (21). Local direct invasion of strap muscles and trachea is characteristic of the more aggressive tumors (22). Resectability depends on this feature, and death may be caused by local invasion and airway obstruction. The "minimally invasive" variant has a far better prognosis than the highly invasive variant.

Follicular carcinomas tend to invade locally and metastasize distantly, rather than to local nodes, and are especially prone to metastasize to bone or lung. In one series (12), one-half had metastasized at the time the diagnosis was originally established. Bony metastases are usually osteolytic, rarely osteoblastic, and the alkaline phosphatase level is rarely elevated. The tumor and metastases often retain an ability to accumulate and hold iodide, and are therefore usually susceptible to treatment with RAI. Indeed, some metastatic tumors synthesize thyroid hormone in normal or even excessive amounts. RAI therapy, as discussed below, improves survival in these patients (21).
Occasionally the primary lesion of a follicular tumor appears to be entirely benign, but distant metastases are found. Invasion of vessels or the capsule, apart from the metastasis, is the only reliable criterion of malignancy. This variant has been called the "benign metastasizing struma" or malignant adenoma. It has a more prolonged course than do other varieties of follicular tumor, and is the type that has offered the best opportunity for the therapeutic use of 131-I. A subset of thyroid carcinomas which have a histologic picture of islands of cells -thus "insular" -has been identified (23). These tumors often look like anaplastic cancers, but sometimes are able to concentrate 131-I and thus are amenable to this treatment. Whether these are properly considered a variety of follicular cancer is uncertain. The important message is that the histology in this instance does not reliably predict the utility of 131-I treatment, suggesting that all patients with thyroid cancer should at some point be studied to determine whether 131-I treatment is possible. The net extra mortality attributable to follicular cancer in the 10 -15 years after diagnosis is 30-50% (12,14,16). Of the patients dying from the lesion, three-fourths do so from the effect of distant metastases and the remainder from locally invasive disease.

Hürthle cell tumors are histologically distinct from other follicular tumors, but they pursue a similar course. They tend to invade and metastasize locally and have a strong propensity to recur after surgery. The course tends to be prolonged. These carcinomas often do not accumulate 131-I. However, in a large survey, Caplan et al (23) found that 4.4% of Hürthle cell neoplasms were hot on scan and 8.9% were "warm". Serum TG levels may be normal or elevated. Cheung et al recently studied the presence of ret/PTC gene rearrangements in Hürthle cell tumors and found that many expressed ret/PTC, and also had other evidence of a papillary cancer origin, including focal nuclear hypochromasia, grooves, and nuclear inclusions. Tumors with the ret/PTC gene rearrangement tended to have lymph node metastases, rather than hematogenous spread. Thus Hürthle cell tumors can be classified into Hürthle cell adenomas, Hürthle cell carcinomas, and Hürthle cell papillary thyroid carcinoma (24).

CHOICE OF OPERATIVE PROCEDURE
Surgical treatment often simultaneously finishes the diagnostic work-up, and initiates therapy. Which operative procedure is indicated when FNA is suspicious or indicative of cancer? (Table 1)

In FNA results classified as suspicious for malignancy have nearly 70-80% chance to be malignant, while an FNA indicative of papillary thyroid cancer is almost always true positive at final histology. Thus, we recommend total (or near-total) thyroidectomy as the initial surgical procedure in these categories, regardless of the size of the nodule. "Near-total" thyroidectomy refers to a procedure which intentionally leaves small portions of thyroid tissue near parathyroid glands or at the entry of the recurrent nerve into the larynx, and is associated with a reduction in possibility of hypoparathyroidism and nerve damage. It is frequently used when post-operative 131-I ablation of residual thyroid tissue is intended.

Some authors prefer lobectomy with frozen section examination in cases when the FNA reveals follicular"neoplasm" (the term implying a new abnormal growth, but not declaring its malignant potential). It must be noted that frozen section carries a significant rate of false negative diagnosis, compared to final histology from paraffin sections. If the diagnosis is positive at final histology, a second operation for completion is generally recommended if lobectomy or sub-total thyroidectomy was initially performed. For these reasons, we prefer total (or near-total) thyroidectomy in these cases.

Table 1 **Suggested Surgical Procedures in Thyroid Cancer**

TYPE	Clinical Class+	OPERATION
Papillary, Follicular	I, <1cm	Lobectomy +/- contralateral STT* (if a < 1cm tumor is detected in a resected specimen, do not reoperate)
Papillary, Follicular	1cm, >1cm, or multicentric, or post-irradiation	NTT** or TT , assessment of possible nodes, primarily in the central compartment
Papillary, Follicular	II,+ neck nodes by US or FNA pre-op, or at operation	NTT + MND***
Papillary, Follicular	III	Resection without mutilation
Papillary, Follicular	IV	Resection without mutilation

TT = intended total thyroidectomy; * STT = Subtotal thyroidectomy; ** NTT = Near-total thyroidectomy; *** MND = Modified neck dissection; +for Clinical Class, see Table 3

Among patients with papillary cancer within the gland, some will have cervical lymph node involvement and others will have no obvious spread. The utility of prophylactic central neck dissection is controversial. Some authoritative centers are in favour, but others, including the authors of this chapter, prefer to perform central neck dissection only when there is a preoperative evidence of lymph node metastases at US, or intraoperative evidence. The same attitude seems indicated for lymph node dissection of other node chains. Whenever a patient treated with lobectomy is found to have a cancer at final histology (sometimes unexpected), the question arises, whether to perform completion thyroidectomy? The indication of several guidelines (25) are in favour of completion thyroidectomy, with the exception of patients with unifocal, small, intrathyroidal, papillary thyroid cancers without evidence of lymph node metastases.

The approach proposed here, is based on several observations. Multicentric involvement is reported to range from 25 to 90%. The wide variation of multicentricity (or intraglandular dissemination) can be explained in part by the finding that the incidence of multicentricity is doubled if one does whole gland histologic sections. There is little or no relationship between the size of a solitary nodule and the incidence of intraglandular dissemination, but an increasing degree of histologic malignancy is associated with the frequency of dissemination. Many extensive studies including those of De Groot et al (26), Mazzaferri et al (18), and Samaan et al (27) supported this procedure. Hay et al. evaluated the efficacy of different surgical approaches to treatment of patients with low risk papillary carcinoma at the Mayo Clinic and concluded that more extensive surgery was not associated with lower case specific mortality rates, but was associated with a lower risk of local regional recurrence. Their data supports the use of bilateral resection as the preferable initial surgical approach (28). Total thyroidectomy carries an increased risk of hypoparathyroidism, recurrent nerve damage, and the necessity for tracheostomy (29). Accidental unilateral nerve damage may reach 5%, but fortunately bilateral injury is rare (30). All surgeons attempt to preserve those parathyroid glands that can be observed and spared, and an attempt is typically made to transplant resected glands into the sternocleidomastoid muscles. Reports range from 1 to a 25% incidence of hypoparathyroidism after total thyroidectomy (15, 31).

TUMOR STAGING AFTER SURGERY

Tumor staging, intended to predict the risk of death or recurrence and guide further therapy, can best be done after initial surgical treatment. The most used staging system is the TNM Staging system which combines simplicity with rather good predictive power (Table 2). Several other staging systems have been developed. The Clinical Class system (Table 3) developed at the University of Chicago classified tumors only on the extent of disease (32), but was found to predict outcome.

Table 2

TNM System of Tumor description and staging developed by the AJCC and UICC

T1	Tumor diameter 2 cm or smaller
T2	Primary tumor diameter >2 to 4 cm
T3	Primary tumor diameter >4 cm limited to the thyroid or with minimal extrathyroidal extension
$T4_a$	Tumor of any size extending beyond the thyroid capsule to invade subcutaneous soft tissues, larynx, trachea, esophagus, or recurrent laryngeal nerve
$T4_b$	Tumor invades prevertebral fascia or encases carotid artery or mediastinal vessels
TX	Primary tumor size unknown, but without extrathyroidal invasion
N0	No metastatic nodes
$N1_a$	Metastases to level VI (pretracheal, paratracheal, and prelaryngeal/Delphian lymph nodes)
$N1_b$	Metastasis to unilateral, bilateral, contralateral cervical or superior mediastinal nodes
NX	Nodes not assessed at surgery
M0	No distant metastases
M1	Distant metastases
MX	Distant metastases not assessed

Stages

	Patient age <45 years	Patient age 45 years or older
Stage I	Any T, any N, M0	T1, N0, M0
Stage II	Any T, any N, M1	T2, N0, M0
Stage III		T3, N0, M0
		T1, $N1_a$, M0
		T2, $N1_a$, M0
		T3, $N1_a$, M0
Stage IVA		$T4_a$, N0, M0
		$T4_a$, $N1_a$, M0
		T1, $N1_b$, M0
		T2, $N1_b$, M0
		T3, $N1_b$, N0
		$T4_a$, $N1_b$, M0
Stage IVB		$T4_b$, Any N, M0
Stage IVC		Any T, Any N, M1

Table 3- Clinical Class description-
I- Intrathyroidal tumor
II-Positive neck nodes
III- Fixed nodes or invasive tumor in the neck
IV- Distant metastases

Several systems are modified to include known risk factors including age, sex, histology, or genetic analysis. The EORTC classification proposed by the European Thyroid Association is based on age, sex, histology, invasion, and metastases (33). The modified

AMES classification includes data on age, extent and size of primary, distant metastases, and DNA ploidy (34). MACIS includes data on age, invasion, metastases, size, and completeness of surgery (35). All of the systems, reviewed by Wong et al (36), appear to be effective in categorizing patients into largely similar low and high risk groups. Invasive disease, metastases, age over 45, and tumor size >4 cm are features placing patients into the high-risk category.

Most recently groups have recently established new criteria for delayed risk assessment based on pathological features combined with clinical features and with the response to initial therapy. Patients in apparent complete remission at follow-up after initial treatment may be defined as low risk, regardless of the initial risk stratification obtained soon after surgery (37). An Italian study (38) assigned patients to low or high risk group at the moment of the first evaluation done 8-12 months after surgery and radioiodine ablation (if performed). Patients free of disease (negative neck US, undetectable basal and stimulated serum TG and no other evidence of disease) were classified at low risk. Patients with any evidence of persistent disease (including detectable TG) were considered at high risk of recurrence. The authors demonstrated that nearly half of the patients could be shifted from the high risk category (at the time of surgery) to the low risk category. The system was named **Delayed Risk Stratification (DRS).** One advantage of these delayed risk stratification systems is that they give an estimate of the risk of recurrence which is not considered in the TNM classification. Whether these systems actually alter therapeutic plans, which naturally evolve as treatment progresses, is uncertain.

TSH SUPPRESSIVE/REPLACEMENT THERAPY
After operation all patients are kept on TSH-suppressive thyroid hormone therapy with l-thyroxine.

Individuals with known cancer receive therapy aimed at a TSH around 0.1 µU/ml. Pushing TSH below this level has not been associated with better outcome, while over-suppression has been associated with more frequent side effects from clinical or subclinical hyperthyroidism, which is often partially mitigated by beta-blockers. Patients who are considered free of disease, have their replacement lowered to provide a TSH in the low-normal range,

RAI 131-I ABLATION
Most patients who have had a "total" thyroidectomy, and all patients who have had a subtotal resection, will have some functioning thyroid tissue remaining in the normal position after surgery, and will thus be candidates for 131-I ablation. This is done to remove any possible residual tumor in the thyroid bed (thyroid ablation), to make subsequent scans and TG assays more interpretable, and (hopefully) to kill tumor cells elsewhere (adjuvant therapy). There is no unanimity regarding the use of postoperative 131-I ablation in Stage I tumors, since absolutely convincing evidence of its value is lacking (15, 39). But for all patients with papillary and follicular cancers as a group, 131-I ablation correlates with improved survival (13). Our data demonstrated that postoperative 131-I ablation correlated with decreased recurrences for all patients with papillary cancers

over 1 cm in size. Samaan et al (27), in a review of 1599 patients, observed that 131-I treatment was the most powerful indicator for disease-free survival.

Ablation after total thyroidectomy can be accomplished in most instances by one dose of 30 mCi (1.1 GBq) 131-I, giving the patients about 10 whole body rads (40). In our practice 80% of patients are ablated successfully with one dose of 30mCi, and the remainder require repeat therapy at the time of their second scan. Other clinicians find this dose insufficient, and give 50-150 mCi (1.85- 5.55 GB) as an inpatient treatment where regulations mandate. In part this difference may depend upon the surgeon, since small remnants of residual thyroid are more easily ablated than large amounts of residual tissue. Low dose (30 mCi) ablation of thyroid tissue after near-total thyroidectomy was recently reviewed by Roos et al. Surveying many studies, they concluded that 30 mCi was as effective as larger doses in inducing ablation, and since it could be administered without hospitalizing the patient, was an appropriate treatment (41). It also minimizes radiation exposure, and damage to the salivary glands. Doses of 100 mCi (3.7 GB) may provide more certain ablation with one dose (although at the expense of greater patient radiation) but there is little difference between ablation rates with doses of 30-75 mCi. There is no data proving that one method or the other provides superior results in terms of survival. We do not routinely use ablation in patients under age 21 with tumors under 1 cm. Patients with tumors above this size, older patients, or those with multicentricity, positive cervical lymph node metastases or a history of neck irradiation are advised to take 131-I. This practice, followed in many clinics, conflicts with some guidelines, as noted below. It has, not surprisingly, been difficult to prove that the addition of RAI ablation reduces mortality in low-risk papillary thyroid cancer, which already has a 20 year survival rate of >95%. However the treatment makes follow-up more precise and reliable by the absence of residual thyroid tissue on scans and ultrasound, by a TG that should be at or below the limit of detectability, and the reassurance to the patient that the tumor is gone. And there are effectively no reported adverse effects of a 30 mCi dose of RAI in the absence of pregnancy.

The indications for thyroid ablation, based on levels of evidence have been detailed in recent ATA guidelines (25). Three groups of patients are identified, one (at very low risk of recurrence) in which thyroid ablation is felt not indicated due to the lack of evidence of benefit; a second group where the benefit, if any, are not evidence based. In this group, ablation was suggested in selected cases according to the judgement of the treating physician. Finally, a third group, including high risk patients, in which ablation has a strong indication based on good evidence that it may reduce cancer recurrence and possibly deaths.

Irrespective of the protocol and the dose used for ablation, there is always a subgroup of about 20% of patients that will not be successfully ablated with the first RAI course. The factors associated with ablation failure are not fully understood. Ablation failure does not correlate precisely with the dose, with the levels of TSH stimulation, the amount of thyroid residue or the level of urinary iodine excretion (42). In particular, it is not certain whether the use of doses higher than 3.70 GBq (100 mCi) would result in any additional benefit, or whether there is a 'stunning' effect of a diagnostic dose of 131-I on the subsequent ablation rate, although unlikely to occur. A retrospective analysis was performed of all patients (n=389) with well-differentiated thyroid cancer treated at our institution between 1992 and 2001. The therapeutic dose was the only variable found to be associated with success (odds ratio, 1.96 per 1.85 GBq (50 mCi) increment). Our results confirm the presence of a significant percentage of ablation failures (24.4%) despite the use of high ablative doses 3.70-7.40 GBq (100-200 mCi). Higher therapeutic doses are associated with higher rates of successful ablation, even when administered to patients with more advanced stages. Higher diagnostic doses were not associated with higher rates of ablation failure. (43).

The utility of radioactive iodide treatment of patients with papillary and follicular cancer was recently reviewed in a series of articles by Wartofsky, Sherman, and Schlumberger and their associates. Schlumberger concludes that routine radioactive iodide ablation is not indicated in patients with differentiated thyroid carcinomas of less than 1.5 cm in diameter, and advocates restricting RAI ablation to patients with poor prognostic indicators for relapse or death (44). Wartofsky points out a secondary benefit of postoperative low dose 131-I ablation in that, for many patients, it provides a high degree of certainty and peace of mind when subsequent scans are negative and TG is undetectable. Another argument for radioactive iodide ablation and early detection of any recurrence is the data presented by several groups, including Schlumberger and colleagues, that there is a reciprocal relationship between the success of cancer therapy and the size and duration of the lesions.

In patients with TNM Stage II to IV disease, we proceed to destroy all residual thyroid and to treat demonstrable metastases if they can be induced to take up enough 131-I. Use of 131-I therapy is investigated in these patients, regardless of the histologic characteristics of the resected lesion, although significant uptake less frequently is found in Hürthle tumors (23,45) or in patients with anaplastic lesions.

PREPARATION FOR 131-I ABLATION

For many years the standard approach has been to induce hypothyroidism prior to the ablative dose in order to raise TSH to approximately 25-30 uU/ml or greater and stimulate uptake of RAI in residual thyroid or tumor. This may be done by simply leaving the patient without T4 therapy for 3 weeks post op, or at any time. Alternatively patients can be given thyroid hormone suppressive therapy for 6 weeks or so after operation, so that any malignant cells disseminated at the time of thyroidectomy will not be stimulated by TSH. The value of this approach is admittedly unknown. Patients then receive 25 µg L-T3 bid for 3-6 weeks, and therapy is then stopped for 2 weeks to allow endogenous TSH (which may reach 20-60 µU/ml) to stimulate uptake of the 131-I by the remaining fragments of thyroid tissue or metastatic lesions in the neck or elsewhere before proceeding with 131-I therapy. These procedures can induce severe hypothyroidism just before scanning, and this is a significant problem and hazard.

An alternative for the initial ablation or later follow-up is the "half-dose" protocol (46). Half the usual dose of thyroxine is given for six weeks. TSH is tested in the fifth week, and if over 20 uU/ml, scanning is done in the sixth week, or preparation is prolonged if needed. On this protocol patients usually feel quasi-normal and conduct normal activities, in contrast to their function during total hormone withdrawal. On the half-dose protocol, fT4 falls to just below normal, and TSH on average reaches about 60uU/ml in the sixth week. Patients who start with TSH below 0.1 uU/ml may take longer to reach a satisfactory level for Tg testing, which is generally considered to be with TSH at least 30 uU/ml.

Many physicians find it useful to have the patient follow a low iodine diet for 2 weeks prior to the planned treatment in an effort to boost RAIU in the remant or tumor.

Stimulation with Recombinant human TSH --During induced hypothyroidism, patients may experience a wide range of hypothyroid signs and symptoms which may be severe and may result in a substantial impairment of the patients' lives and ability to drive and to work, and occasional tumor growth. Recombinant human TSH (Thyrogen®) has been developed to meet the need for safe, adequate exogenous TSH stimulation in patients with papillary and follicular thyroid carcinoma. The TG level reached after rhTSH stimulation is generally lower than that obtained after thyroid hormone withdrawal, and RAI uptakes in patients undergoing hormone withdrawal are higher, indicating that withdrawal provides a much greater and more prolonged stimulus to thyroid or tumor tissue. However, the diagnostic results are nearly equal. Quality of life is better using rhTSH preparation than during hypothyroidism induced by total thyroid hormone withdrawal, and side effects are minimal. Clinical trials have shown that rhTSH is an effective and safe alternative to thyroid hormone withdrawal during the post-surgical follow-up of papillary and follicular thyroid cancer, although not as sensitive as scanning after hormone withdrawal in some patients. Another factor to consider is the cost, which is roughly $ 2000 per treatment, although for the majority of patients in the USA this is covered by insurance. A few patients have been reported with metastases demonstrated on withdrawal scans that were not evident on rhTSH scans (47). A more prolonged stimulation of residual tissue may be necessary in some instances. It has been found that rhTSH administration induces a reduction of serum vascular endothelial growth factor, even in the absence of thyroid tissue (48). The clinical significance of this observation, if any, is unknown, but it does imply possible action of rhTSH on receptors other than in thyroid tissue. Use of rhTSH in managing thyroid cancer has recently been extensively reviewed (49). Thanks to many studies confirming the properties of rhTSH in stimulating iodine uptake and TG production, rhTSH is now considered an accepted alternative method of preparation for both thyroid ablation and post-surgical follow-up in patients with any form of differentiated thyroid cancer. After any planned period of dietary iodine restriction, two doses of rhTSH are given when the patient is on replacement treatment, and TG assay, dosing for scan or treatment is done 24 hours after the second injection, and scans are done 48-72 hours later.

Diagnostic scans before first ablation are no longer routinely indicated according to several groups and ATA guidelines (25), based on the evidence that they do not offer additional information compared to the post-therapy scan and based on the possibility of stunning. However some authors point out that pre-ablation or pre-therapy scans can reveal unknown disease that may indicate increased treatment dose requirement, or lack of iodide uptake due to non-functioning or eradicated tumor tissue, which would preclude doing a treatment, or lack of uptake due to unexpected high iodine intake by the patient. If one intends to scan, the usual scanning dose should be no higher than 1-2 mCi 131-I, which has not been shown to induce stunning. 123-I can also be used to reduce radiation, but has a short half-life. Scans should be read at 48 or 72 hours, when body background has diminished. If TSH is sufficiently elevated the initial scan can reveal distant metastases as well as residual thyroid gland. If large thyroid tissue remnants are present, TSH may not become very elevated after hormone withdrawal, but will do so after the first ablation dose. Excess iodine intake in any form, including contrast studies, may suppress RAIU for weeks and should be considered, and avoided,

Some physicians proceed without prior scanning directly to 131-I ablation 2-4 weeks after surgery and perform a post-therapy scan 5-7 days later. Presumed benefits of this approach are patient convenience, less expense, and avoidance of possible thyroid "stunning" by the scan dose. In fact, as noted above stunning has not been demonstrated with the 2mCi 131-I dose. Arguments for doing a pre-ablation scan include finding out the actual percent uptake of the treatment dose in the neck and elsewhere to be considered when counselling about radiation safety required isolation periods, establishing if in fact there is uptake, and recognizing disease that may dictate a larger initial dose. The final word on these different approaches is not in.

It is useful to measure urinary iodine prior to scan or treatment since if elevated significantly (above 500ug/day, especially if >1mg/day) iodine uptake in thyroid or tumor may be suppressed.

Patients with Class I and in many with disease who are under age 45 are given 30 mCi as an out-patient treatment. Older Patients with Class II, III or IV disease are given doses of 75-100 mCi, in some states necessitating inpatient treatment. A post-therapy whole body scans should be mandatory 5-7 days after the ablative dose of 131-I (or after therapeutic doses), since occasionally unsuspected metastasis may be visualized on scans at this time changing the stage of disease and modifying the risk of reoccurrence or death. A stimulated baseline serum TG is always measured at the time of 131-I therapy. At 24 hours after initial ablative treatment, we replace hormone therapy at the prior dose.

OPTIONS IN FOLLOW-UP SCANS AND TREATMENT-INCLUDING RECENTLY DESCRIBED VARIATIONS

After surgery and thyroid ablation, the first important time for follow-up is between 8 and 12 months after initial treatment. At this time we want to understand whether the patients have evidence of complete remission or some evidence of persistent or recurrent disease. In the past, the conventional preparation for follow-up was to obtain a diagnostic total body scan with 131-I after induction of hypothyroidism, with the same methodology as described for ablation, in order to stimulate uptake of 131-I by residual thyroid tissue or tumor cells and production of TG. In recent years it has become common to omit the diagnostic scans after initial ablation, at least in patients deemed to be at low risk, and relying on measurement of stimulated (after rhTSH administration) serum TG when anti-Tg antibodies are negative (25). In patients known to have residual disease because of elevated baseline TG or ultrasound evidence of metastatic lymph nodes, therapeutic 131-I is often given without preliminary scanning. In several large series, it was demonstrated that at this time of the follow-up, more than 80% of the patients will have evidence of complete remission (negative neck US and undetectable stimulated serum TG levels). These patients do not require additional tests or imaging and their suppressive hormone therapy should be shifted to replacement targeting serum TSH in the low-normal range. In subsequent years, the chance of these patients to have a recurrence is extremely low (<1%) and thus their follow up should be based on basal TG measurement and neck US once a year. On the contrary, when neck US is positive for local disease, or the basal or stimulated TG is elevated the patient should be screened for the localization of the disease and treated accordingly. Exactly what TG level is "elevated" is a shifting target, and depends on the local assay and experience. TG >2 ng/ml after rhTSH or withdrawal of hormone has been one standard. Possibly, with assays now accurate below 0.1ng/ml, a basal or suppressed TG > 0.5-1ng may be considered abnormal. Whether this approach, which essentially eliminates follow-up WB scans in low risk patients, provides satisfactory long-term outcome, is yet to be determined.

FOLLOW -UP TREATMENT BASED ON TG ASSAYS

As assays for thyroglobulin (TG) have become more sensitive and reliable, measurement of TG assumes more and more importance in determining the management of patients followed after thyroidectomy and radioactive iodide ablation treatment for thyroid cancer. Serum TG levels, in the absence of antibodies interfering in the assay, correlate well with tumor burden, although detectable tumor can exist even in the presence of negative TG assays in individuals who are on suppressive doses of thyroid hormone (50). It is proposed that diagnostic 131-I whole body scans can be avoided in patients with undetectable levels of stimulated TG after initial ablation, and that the patients can be monitored with clinical examination, ultrasound, and serial TG measurements on thyroxine treatment during the subsequent follow-up

However, some concerns with this approach have been noted. Mazzaferri and Kloos (51) retrospectively studied 107 patients who were "clinically free of disease" and had undetectable or very low serum TG levels during thyroid hormone therapy. The TG levels on treatment were all 1 ng/ml or less, and 95% were under 0.5 ng/ml in their assay, which was a commercial (Nichols Institute) chemoluminescent antibody assay. In response to the administration of two doses of recombinant TSH and assay of TG on samples taken on the fifth day, 20% were found to have a TG value above 2, with values ranging up to 18 ng/m, and many of these patients ended up with additional 131-I therapy. However, the authors found that diagnostic, pre-ablation radioactive iodide whole body scans often failed to localize the source of the elevated TG, which was found only in post-therapy scans or by other imaging methods. This study suggests that even with a TG level below 1 while on replacement therapy, persistent disease may sometimes be present and be detected by stimulation using recombinant TSH or thyroid hormone withdrawal.

Wartofsky (52, 53) comments on these studies and supports the idea that TG testing, both on suppression and after TSH stimulation, can help in determining therapy. He suggests that, in patients with a serum TG <0.5ng/ml on suppression, and in a low risk category, that stimulation by recombinant TSH and measurement of TG, rather than scanning, is satisfactory. If the TG remains <1, the patients can be evaluated annually with such a stimulation test. In patients with slightly higher TGs, up to 2, he suggests measuring a recombinant TSH stimulated TG, and scanning. In patients with higher TGs, he suggests that thyroid hormone withdrawal and radioactive iodide treatment, without initial scanning, may be appropriate. In a study done by the rhTSH-Stimulated Thyroglobulin Study Group (54) and published in 2002, a cut off level of 1 ng/ml for stimulated TG was taken as the safe level for patients with low risk. This group would presumably be monitored by repeat rhTSH stimulated TG assays rather than scans. It is of interest that in this study 14 of the patients with stimulated TG <2ng/ml underwent isotope scanning and 9 were positive. Five had uptake outside the thyroid bed. This group suggests that patients with stimulated TG above 2 would have subsequent thyroid hormone withdrawal and possible 131-I therapy without scanning. A recent "consensus" statement by a group of thyroidologists also supports the categorization of patients into high and low risk groups, and use of TG as described above for following low risk patients (55). Whether this approach, with omission of whole body scans, has any adverse effect on long term outcome is not yet known.

Another option coming "on-line" is the use of ultra-sensitive TG assays (in patients without anti-TG antibodies) since the information appears to partially substitute for rhTSH stimulated TG assays. Several reports indicate (56) that, when using assays with detectability to 0.1ng/ml, an undetectable TG is associated with complete remission in almost all case and may safely be substituted for a TG stimulation test. Detectable values, even if under 0.5ng/nil, probably should be supplemented by a stimulated TG.

TREATMENT USING EMPIRICALLY DETERMINED DOSES OF 100- 150MCI FOR METASTATIC DISEASE

Patients who have significant uptake of 131-I in distant metastases (usually above 0.5% of the tracer) are given 150-250 mCi 131-I. This dose can be tolerated without acute radiation sickness, and is below the level that would promote pulmonary fibrosis if diffuse pulmonary metastases are present, unless uptake in the lungs exceeds 50% (see below). Although use of these empirically derived doses is the most common practice, some centers do careful dosimetry with a tracer dose of 131-I prior to therapy, in order to judge the appropriate, or maximal safe, dose. This requires 2-5 days of observation. The methodology and results have been recently discussed (57). Whether administration of maximally large individual doses is more effective than use of somewhat smaller doses of 131-I has not been established. In perhaps four-fifths of patients accumulating 131-I, it is possible to administer a dose of RAI that should be useful in destroying tumor. For normal thyroid tissue 10,000-15,000 rads is destructive, and a dose of 20,000 rads or more is probably needed for therapy of cancer. Assuming, for example, a standard 150 mCi 131-I dose, and delivery to tumor of about 100 rads per micro Curie retained per gram, a 1% tumor uptake distributed through 10 g of metastatic tissue could provide an effective treatment.

Some groups have attempted to measure tumor volume by use of quantitative I-124 PET scanning if available (58). The effective half-life can be determined from serial counts of the tracer over the metastasis. If 10 g of tumor in the neck accumulated 1% of a 150 mCi dose, and isotope turnover in the tumor was extremely slow, the radiation dose might be as follows: Rads $= 74 \times 0.19 \times 150,000 \times 0.01 \times 6/10 = 12,654$ rads.

The question of whether a sub-cancericidal doses should be delivered in patients with low levels of tumor isotope accumulation needs further investigation, since radiobiological studies suggest that radiation could preferentially spare the more radio resistant cells, ultimately leaving a more lethal tumor while cumulative exposure to the bone marrow and salivary glands may reach morbidity inducing levels. It may be possible to give conventional x-ray therapy after 131-I in those instances in which 131-I uptake is present but the total dose delivered to the metastasis is less than adequate (59). This procedure may provide another therapeutic approach to the thyroid cancer patient, but it has not yet been given adequate trial. Maxon et al (60) report that radiation doses of at least 30,000 rads for thyroid ablation, and 8,000 for therapy to metastasis, improve the rate of response.

It is useful to do a scintiscan on patients who have received therapeutic doses of 131-I at 5 -7days following the treatment, thus using the treatment dose as a more powerful and sensitive scanning dose. While often offering no new information (which may be reassuring to the patrient), this may also reveal unsuspected metastasis, especially in younger patients who have previously had 131-I treatment. Fatourechi et al found that 13% of follow-up scans demonstrated abnormal foci of uptake not seen on diagnostic scans, and changed management in 9% of their patients (45, 61).

The 131-I treatment cycle is repeated at 24-52 weeks, as long as there is no evidence of systemic radiation damage, and as long as the metastases continue to accumulate iodide. The total cumulative 131-I dosage may vary from 150 to (rarely) 2,000 mCi (74GB). Both papillary and follicular cancers respond to 131-I therapy. Small metastases from papillary cancer, especially if functional in the lungs but not large enough to be visualized on X-ray, are typically cured. Follicular tumors often have relatively few metastases and high uptake, thus seem ideal targets for therapy. However portions of the metastases, especially in bone, often appear to be resistant and finally continue growth despite 131-I treatment. Nevertheless 131-I therapy is beneficial even in advanced and aggressive tumors. Pelikan et al report their experience on the use of radioactive iodide in treating advanced differentiated thyroid carcinoma and report that up to 50% of patients who have distant metastases can be cured by 131-I therapy (62). Aggressive high dose radioiodine therapy has been advocated for treatment of advanced differentiated thyroid cancer by Menzel and colleagues. These physicians gave repeated doses of 300 mCi (11.1 GBq 131-I) with mean accumulated total activities of, on average, 55 GBq (1500 mCi) per patient. Repetitive high dose therapy appeared beneficial in the majority of patients with papillary carcinoma, but the majority of follicular thyroid cancer patients had progressive disease despite treatment (63).

The National Thyroid Cancer Treatment Cooperative Study Registry Group recently evaluated the therapy of high risk papillary and non-Hürthle cell follicular thyroid carcinoma. The study confirmed the utility and benefit of radioactive iodide therapy to reduce recurrence and cancer-specific mortality among patients in the high risk group (64). Pittas et al. (65) reviewed an extensive series of 146 patients with documented bone metastasis from thyroid carcinoma seen at Memorial Sloan Kettering in New York City. Bone metastases were most common in vertebrae, pelvis, ribs, and femur, and multiple lesions were present in more than half the cases. Overall ten year survival rate was 35%, and from diagnosis of initial bone metastasis, 10 year survival was 13%. Favorable prognostic signs for survival included radioiodine uptake by the metastases and absence of non-osseous metastases. Hürthle cell cancers had a favorable response to treatment, rather surprisingly, whereas undifferentiated thyroid tumors fared the worst.

Arterial embolization has been combined with radioactive iodide treatment for management of large bone metastasis from differentiated thyroid carcinoma with apparent improvement in effect over the use of radioactive iodide alone. In the study by VanTol et al, (66) embolization was not accompanied by any severe complications.

rhTSH is now available for routine use except for high-risk patients, and allows 131-I therapy without induction of hypothyroidism (67). This can increase acceptance of scanning and therefore increase the frequency of diagnostic procedures. Iodide depletion by dietary control and diuresis, including furosemide or mannitol administration, can also double the fractional uptake of 131-I in metastases (68, 69). Finally, when the diagnostic scan shows no 131-I uptake, even with TSH, the potential benefits from this mode of therapy have probably been exhausted. However, before giving up on 131-I therapy, some authors suggest using empiric 100-150mCi doses of 131-I and obtaining a post-therapy scan, which in some cases may show areas of uptake not seen in the diagnostic scan (see below).

HIGH DOSE RAI THERAPY FOR INVASIVE OR METASTATIC DISEASE

Ablation of thyroid tumors of follicular cell origin with high doses of RAI is a common procedure. Initially heralded as a panacea, it has proven otherwise, although useful.

Efficacy and morbidity of high activity 131-I therapy was assessed in 38 patients with locally advanced or metastatic differentiated thyroid cancer (16 follicular, 20 papillary, one Hürthle cell, one insular) who were treated with high activity radioiodine therapy (9 GBq [250 mCi]) as the cancers had previously not responded to standard activities of 5.5 GBq (150 mCi). After high activity treatment, 9.7% of patients suffered grade 3 and 3.2% suffered grade 4 WHO hematological toxicity. Significant salivary gland morbidity was observed (30% dry mouth, 27% salivary swelling). In this study repeated treatment with high activity (9 GBq) in patients with advanced differentiated thyroid carcinoma appeared to be of no apparent benefit but led to late morbidity (359). However, other investigators have differing results. A retrospective analysis was conducted on 124 differentiated thyroid cancer patients who underwent dosimetric evaluation over a period of 15 years. One hundred four RAI treatments were performed. A complete response at metastatic deposits was attained with absorbed doses of >100Gy. No permanent BM suppression was observed in patients who received absorbed doses of<3Gy to BM. The maximum administered dose was 38.5 GBq (1,040 mCi) with the BM dose limitation. Dosimetry-guided RAI treatment allowed administration of the maximum possible RAI dose to achieve the maximum therapeutic benefit. Estimation of tumor dose rates helped to determine the curative versus the palliative intent of the therapy (71).

131-I THERAPY WITH "NEGATIVE" SCANS

In some patients tracer studies fail to show uptake, but serum TG is elevated (with or without stimulation). Some investigators recommend treating these individuals with large doses of 131-I (100-150 mCi) and report that tumor uptake can be visualized after treatment, and that serum TG may fall (72, 73). The clinical efficacy of this approach is not known. In a few cases reported by Schlumberger et al. (74) and Pineda et al. (75) TG became undetectable, which clearly was a striking and hopeful result. As of this date, there is no data demonstrating that this treatment approach improves prognosis (377).
 The utility of radioactive iodide treatment of patients with papillary and follicular cancer was recently reviewed in a series of articles by Wartofsky, Sherman, and Schlumberger and their associates (44). Sherman and Gopal analysed the use of 100 mCi doses of 131-I for treatment of scan-negative TG-positive patients and conclude that this must, at this point, be considered an experimental procedure of uncertain benefit. They argue against its use in young patients with elevated although apparently stable TG values and without radiographic evidence of disease. Fatourechi et al. (77) analysed results of this

treatment in a series of patients treated at the Mayo Clinic and concluded that it rarely produced significant effect, although it possibly helped stabilize disease in patients with micro metastases in the lung. It is clearly ineffective in patients who have metastases large enough to be detected on chest X-ray or CAT. Wartofsky et al. (44) suggest that, rather than initial treatment with 131-I of patients who are scan negative and TG-positive, thorough imaging studies are appropriate. These might include a CAT scan of the chest, an MRI of the neck, 99mTc-MIBI, 18-fluorine fluorodeoxyglucose PET scanning, 99mTc-tetrafosmin, or 201TI thallium. Localization of malignant tissue by any of these means may allow surgical excision or external radiotherapy. This series of articles provides many very useful thoughts on management of difficult patients with recurrent thyroid carcinoma.

MAXIMUM DOSE PROTOCOLS

The therapeutic protocol used at Memorial Hospital in New York, by Maxon (60), and as well at some other centers, has for years been designed to give maximal-tolerable radiation doses to cancer patients (12). The dose is calculated on the basis of prior isotope tracer kinetics. The aim is to give a blood dose of under 200 rads, or less than 120 mCi (4.4 GB) retained at 48 hours, or 80 mCi (30 GB) retained at 48 hours if diffuse lung metastases are present. This method has theoretical advantages since it potentially provides the most cancericidal dose, but the difficulties of calculating the dose and the occasional adverse reactions have so far prevented this method from being generally employed. The dosimetric approach has been carefully reviewed by Van Nostrand et al (55).

RADIATION PRECAUTIONS

Before radiation therapy, female patients should be carefully screened for pregnancy and lactation. Confirmed or possible pregnancy constitutes an absolute contraindication to therapy because of the risk of damage to the fetus. A patient who has ingested many millicuries of 131-I can cause serious radiation contamination, and appropriate precautions must be followed. If less than 30 mCi 131-I is given, it is permissible to have the patient dispose of urine and feces into general sewage in most regulatory jurisdictions. If amounts of 131-I greater than 30 mCi are given, and in some states the patient may need be kept in a private room in the hospital until less than 30 mCi is retained in the body. Urine can be directly disposed in sewage, or can be collected by the patient and stored in bottles behind protective lead shielding. After physical decay, usually after about 6 weeks, it may be discarded in the sewage. Contaminated bedding and utensils should be stored for 10 half-lives (80 days), thoroughly washed, and monitored for residual contamination before being used again. Alternatively, disposable bedding and utensils may be used.

Table 4. Radiation Exposure to Personnel During Care of a Patient Who Has Received 100 mCi 131-I

Distance From Source – e.g The Patient	Reason for Exposure	Rate (mrad/hr)	Allowable Duration of Exposure Permitted on Basis of 0.1Rad/Week
1/2 in.	Direct handling of therapy dose or urine after therapy	136000	None
1 ft.	Giving personal hygiene to treated patient	240	0.5 hr/week
3 ft.	Making the bed, mopping the floor	27	5.0 hr/week
9 ft.	In chair across the room	3	50.0 hr/week allowable exposure cannot be reached

Personnel caring for a patient who has received 131-I therapy are often concerned about exposure to excessive radiation. This is almost never a real problem. Isotope can, at a practical level, only be passed from the patient to another person via saliva or urine. Monitoring by means of a portable counter is important in making certain that no person receives more than an allowable radiation dose from the isotope in the patient's body. Table 4 gives a rough estimate of the amount of radiation received while performing ordinary hospital tasks at various distances from a patient who has received 131-I. In general, all ordinary patient care can be performed without hazard. It is best to avoid close contact between hospital personnel and patient during the first 48 hours after therapy because of undue apprehension that may be induced. However, even after doses of up to 100 mCi (3.7 GB), normal personal activities such as eating at the same table, or driving in the same car, carry no risk to others.

The US Nuclear Regulatory Commission has published new guidelines which allow release of patients treated with isotopes from the hospital if the total effective radiation exposure from the treated person to any other individual is not likely to exceed 5mSv (0.5 rads). Grigsby et al (78) found that when using precautions such as those described above in a group of patients given on average about 100mCi 131-I, the exposure to other individuals in their household and to pets did not exceed this level. Guidelines for the optimal radiation protection after treatment with 131-I have been proposed by the American Thyroid Association (79) (WWW.THYROID.ORG) and offer much specific and useful advice.

RADIATION DAMAGE FROM 131-I THERAPY

The use of RAI in large doses is not without hazard. The radiation dose delivered to the whole body, the gonads, or bone marrow is usually assumed to be the same as that of the blood. The blood dose depends on the amount of isotope administered; its distribution space and turnover; the degree of heterogeneity of distribution in the tumor; the uptake, synthesis, and secretion of labelled compound by the tumor; and perhaps other variables. The radiation is usually largely due to inorganic iodide, since little protein bound (PB) 131-I ordinarily appears in the blood. Sometimes tumor destruction is such that much PB131-I appears in the blood and can yield a major fraction of the total whole body radiation dose. As a rough estimate, the blood, gonadal, or bone marrow radiation may be assumed to be 0.3 -1.5 rads/mCi 131-I administered (80), or 45-150 rads per treatment with 100 mCi. The genetic risks are discussed in www.thyroidmanager.org and are not reviewed here. Ordinarily, when 131-I therapy is needed for carcinoma, the necessity of treating the patient outweighs the risks of genetic damage.

Various unwanted effects of radiation may occur in patients receiving large doses of 131-I. Mild radiation sickness is seen. Metastatic deposits or surrounding tissues may become painful over 2-4 weeks from radiation-induced inflamation. Damage to the salivary glands can cause sialadenitis, and xerostomia, and can lead to loss of teeth (81). Increasing salivary flow following treatment may be partially protective. Ovarian function is often temporarily suppressed (82), and if there are pelvic metastases that collect 131-I, the gonads may receive a sterilizing dose. Sperm count may be reduced for months (83). Leukemia occurs with increased frequency in patients who have received large doses of 131-I (usually >600 mCi [22GB]) for cancer (217). Transient or permanent alterations in liver function and lymphoma of the parotid gland have been reported as possible sequelae (85). Pulmonary fibrosis has occurred in patients with functioning lung metastases who have received unusually large doses or who have very active metastases (86). Leukopenia, thrombocytopenia, and anemia are encountered with accumulating doses. A mild effect on the bone marrow is seen with each therapeutic dose, and after several hundred kilocuries, aplastic anemia may develop (87). The hemoglobin level, white cell count, differential count, and platelets should be monitored periodically in order to judge recovery of the marrow between treatments and to prevent excess total radiation damage to the marrow. Large radiation doses may cause transient swelling of metastasis in the brain or spinal canal. Lin et al (88) recently reviewed pregnancies following 131-I treatment of well differentiated thyroid carcinoma among a group of 58 pregnant women and found no evidence of demonstrable adverse effects, but suggest that it would be wise to avoid pregnancy during the first six months after the last administration of 131-I. With the exception of possibly increased rate of miscarriages which may have been due unstable thyroid function at the time of conception, no other adverse effect of radioiodine has been found on the outcome of 2113 pregnancies after radioiodine treatment and on their offspring (34).

Two special complications need be noted. Occasionally withdrawal of hormone suppression, in preparation for isotope therapy, leads to rapid growth of the tumor, and reinstitution may not seem to return the patient to the prior condition. Special care should be taken if metastases are present in areas such as brain or spinal column, where growth could cause serious sequelae. Glucocorticoids are occasionally given prophylactically in an effort to prevent tumor swelling in this situation.

Disseminated pulmonary metastasis can sometimes be eradicated by 131-I, but radiation pneumonitis or fibrosis may be produced and may be fatal (38, 86). On first observation of pulmonary metastases, this therapy should be considered, but no more than 75 mCi (2.9 GB) should ever be deposited in the lungs in one treatment. Progress of the lesion and pulmonary function should be carefully evaluated before and between treatments (89, 90-94). Occasionally patients present with locally advanced papillary thyroid cancer which is not surgically resectable. In some instances preoperative treatment with radioactive iodide sufficiently reduces the extent of the lesion to allow subsequent definitive surgery (94). One of the most informative studies regarding the effects and limitation of 131-I therapy is given by the series of the Institute Gustave-Roussy periodically updated by Schlumberger et al (95). In their most recent publication the authors report on 444 patients treated with 131-I for distant metastases and the results identified three groups of patients with different outcome after therapy: a group very likely to be cured after a few courses of RAI, represented by young patients with micronodular disease, usually in the lung; a second group whose metastases can be stabilized but not cured after more than 600 mCi (22 GB) as cumulative doses and a third group including older patients with macronodular disease, particularly in the bones, who do not respond to RAI and progress rapidly to exitus. It is apparent from this study that, continuing RAI therapy after 600 mCi usually has no benefit.

FOLLOW-UP OF CANCER PATIENTS: THE SERUM TG ASSAY.

After initial ablation patients are given TSH-suppressive doses of l-thyroxine. This therapy as dual aims: to replace the thyroid hormone function and to inhibit the growth of potential residual disease. Two to three months later serum TSH, free thyroid hormones and TG concentrations are measured during l-thyroxine treatment. The results of these tests will disclose whether the l-thyroxine dose is adequate in suppressing TSH levels without inducing thyrotoxicosis, but will give little information on whether the patient is in remission.To this purpose, the most informative follow-up period is at 6-12 months after initial treatment, when the ablative dose of radioiodine should have exerted its effect. At this point, the patients have been already attributed a risk estimate based on the results of the post-ablative WBS and serum TG measurement (96, 97. This information is important at the moment of the new evaluation. If uptake was seen outside the thyroid bed on the post-therapy WBS, the patient must be considered at high risk of recurrence or persistent disease, while if no uptake is seen outside the thyroid bed on the 131-I post-therapy scan, the Patient is considered at low-risk. The 6-12 month evaluation, consists of careful neck ultrasound to detect the lymph node status and serum TG levels (with negative anti-TG) after stimulation with exogenous (better) or endogenous TSH. These tests are considered by many authors as sufficient to confirm complete remission (negative US and undetectable stimulated TG). Others advocate the usefulness of a diagnostic WBS with radioiodine, aimed to ensure that thyroid ablation has been successful and to search for foci of 131-I uptake outside the thyroid bed. However, two independent studies (357, 99) have shown that this diagnostic WBS is almost always negative (depending on criteria for positivity) thus adding very little information to that given by neck US and serum TG measurement.

The result of serum TG measurement is the most sensitive predictor of complete remission or persistent disease (provided that anti-Tg autoantibodies are negative) (100-104). Nearly all patients with local or distant disease have detectable or elevated serum TG levels, while patients in stable remission have undetectable serum TG concentrations. Compared to serum TG measurement, the yield of the diagnostic 131-I WBS is lower. A significant proportion of patients may have an elevation of serum Tg in the presence of a negative diagnostic WBS. A retrospective study by Cailleaux et al. (98) has shown that when serum Tg off therapy is undetectable, routine diagnostic WBS usually does not add any further information on the clinical status of the patient. Similar results have been obtained at the Department of Endocrinology, University of Pisa, (99) in a retrospective series of 315 patients who had undetectable serum Tg off l-thyroxine at the time of the first re-evaluation after thyroid ablation. None of these patients had evidence of disease activity at WBS, and 99.4% were in complete and stable remission after 12 years of follow-up. Only two patients (0.6%) had recurrence of lymph node metastases which were treated with radioiodine therapy. Based on these studies it is possible that in the future the need for 131-I scanning may be dictated by the results of serum TG during hypothyroidism or by rhTSH-stimulation
After this follow up, low-risk patients (those with an undetectable stimulated serum Tg, negative neck US and negative WBS, when performed) are considered as cured and may be followed with periodic serum Tg measurement during l-thyroxine therapy. Thyroxine therapy may be decreased to maintain a low but not suppressed serum TSH concentration (0.1-0.4 µU/ml). The risk of recurrence is in fact so low in these patients (representing more than 80% of the total) that overdosage of l-thyroxine is unjustified.

As noted the problem of antibody interference in the TG assay makes this test unreliable in 10-15% of patients. However another aspect of the antibodies should be remembered. If patients are free of thyroid cancer and the thyroid has been ablated, it appears that the antigenic stimulation necessary to maintain an anti-TG titer is gradually lost, and these antibodies disappear with a 3-6 year half-life (302). Thus, the level of anti-Tg antibodies may be used as a surrogate marker of disease. Other approaches, including the search of Tg mRNA in the blood, have been proposed, but none has entered general clinical practice. Fugazzola et al (106) point out that the combination of TG RIA and TG mRNA assay offer better positive and negative predictive value than TG alone. In some studies TG mRNA analysis has proven much less reliable than serum TG assay (107).

In high risk patients, even if considered cured, suppressive doses of l-thyroxine may be continued for some years, because the risk of relapse is greater. Pujol et al evaluated a series of patients over an average of 95 months and compared those who had TSH values constantly under 0.05 mU/l to those who had all TSH values greater than 1mU/l. A lesser degree of TSH suppression was associated with an increased incidence of relapse, with a shorter average relapse-free survival (108). This observation was not sustained in another study (109. The objective of suppressive therapy in these patients should be to attain a serum TSH level of 0.1 µU/ml or less with normal free T3. In this situation, side effects such as osteoporosis, are not observed (110). Clinical and biochemical evaluation is performed annually. If serum Tg becomes detectable during follow-up, the patient should be evaluated for the presence of disease by neck US, first, and by other imaging if neck ultrasound is negative. Some authors prefer to avoid this procedure and directly give a therapeutic dose of 131-I followed by a post-therapy scan. In the absence of uptake after therapeutic doses of 131-I, any further administration of 131-I is not justified, and the site of Tg production should be sought by other imaging techniques. If 131-I thyroid ablation has not been performed or if the patient has undergone only partial thyroid surgery (subtotal or lobectomy), follow-up should consist of clinical and ultrasound examination and serum Tg measurement. However, in this case, the sensitivity and specificity of serum TG assay is lost. In such patients, any suspicion of persistent or recurrence disease should prompt a completion of the initial treatment with completion thyroidectomy and/or radioiodine ablation.

During follow-up, patients may develop isolated metastases that can be approached surgically. Osseous metastases, especially from follicular cancer, may require radiotherapy or operative procedures for stabilization. Progressive growth of soft tissue or osseous metastases that are not amenable to further suppression with thyroid hormone, 131-I therapy, or radiotherapy should lead to consideration of systemic therapies.

Radiation Therapy, Chemotherapy, Re-differentiation therapy, and use of biological response modifiers such as TKI inhibitors, are discussed elsewhere in this symposium.

REFERENCES

1. Halnan, K 1966. Influence of age and sex on incidence and prognosis of thyroid cancer. Cancer 19:1534.

2. Russel, M, Gilbert, E, Jaeschke, W 1975. Prognostic features of thyroid cancer. A long term follow-up of 68 cases. Cancer 36:553.

3. Rosvoll, R, Winship, T 1965. Thyroid carcinoma and pregnancy. Surg Gynecol Obstet 121:1039.

4. Franssila, K 1975. Prognosis in thyroid carcinoma. Cancer 36:1138.

5. Woolner, L, Lemmon, M, Beahrs, O, Black, B, Keating, F J 1960. Occult papillary carcinoma of the thyroid. Study of 140 cases observed in a 30-year period. J Clin Endocrinol Metab 20:89-113.

6. Passler, C; Prager, G; Scheuba, C; Niederle, BE; Kaserer, K; Zettinig, G; Niederle, B. Follicular variant of papillary thyroid carcinoma: a long-term follow-up. Arch Surg 138:1362-1366,2003.

7. Shattuck TM, Westra WH, Ladenson PW, Arnold A. Independent clonal origins of distinct tumor foci in multifocal papillary thyroid carcinoma. N Engl J Med. 2005, 352:2406-12.

8. McConahey, W, Taylor, W, Gorman, C, Woolner, L Field. Educational Italian Retrospective study of 820 patients treated for papillary carcinoma of the thyroid at the Mayo Clinic between 1946 and 1971. In Andreoli, M; Monaco, F; Robbins, J (eds). Advances in Thyroid Neoplasia: Rome.

9. C. Ceccarelli, F. Pacini, F. Lippi, R. Elisei, M. Arganini, P. Miccoli, A. Pinchera. Thyroid cancer in children and adolescent. Surgery 104:1143, 1988.

10. McDermott, W J, Morgan, W, Hamlin, E J, Cope, O 1954. Cancer of the thyroid. J Clin Endocrinol Metab 14:1336.

11. Schlumberger, M, De Vathaire, F, Travagli, J, et al. 1987. Differentiated thyroid carcinoma in childhood. Long term follow-up of 72 patients. J Clin Endocrinol Metab 65:1088.

12. Cady, B, Sedgwick, C, Meissner, W, Bookwalter, J, Romagosa, V, Werber, J 1976. Changing clinical; pathologic; therapeutic; and survival patterns of differentiated thyroid carcinoma. Ann Surg 184:541.

13. Mazzaferri, E, Young, R 1981. Papillary thyroid carcinoma. A ten year follow-up report of the impact of therapy in 576 patients. Am J Med 70:511.

14. Harwood, J, Clark, O, Dunphy, J 1978. Significance of lymph node metastasis in differentiated thyroid cancer. Am J Surg 136:107.

15. Mazzaferri, E, Young, R, Oertel, J, Kemmerer, W, Page, C 1977. Papillary thyroid carcinoma. The impact of therapy in 576 patients. Medicine 56:171.

16. Terry, J, St John, S, Karkowski, F, al., e 1994. Tall cell papillary thyroid cancer. Incidence and prognosis. Am J Surg 168:459.

17. Burman, K, Ringel, M, Wartofsky, L 1996. Unusual types of thyroid neoplasms.

Endocrinol Metab Clinics North America 25:49-68.

18. Grebe SK, Hay ID. Follicular thyroid cancer. Endocrinol Metab Clin North Am. 1995, 24:761-801.

19. Elisei R, Molinaro E, Agate L, Bottici V, Masserini L, Ceccarelli C, Lippi F, Grasso L, Basolo F, Bevilacqua G, Miccoli P, Di Coscio G, Vitti P, Pacini F, Pinchera A. Are the clinical and pathological features of differentiated thyroid carcinoma really changed over the last 35 years? Study on 4187 patients from a single Italian institution to answer this question. J Clin Endocrinol Metab. 2010, 95:1516-27.

20. Chao, TC; Lin, JD; Chen, MF. Insular carcinoma: Infrequent subtype of thyroid cancer with aggressive clinical course. World J Surg, 2004, 28:393-6.

21. Young, R, Mazzaferri, E, Rahe, A, Dorfman, S 1980. Pure follicular thyroid carcinoma. Impact of therapy in 214 patients. J Nucl Med 21:733.

22. Justin, E, Seabold, J, Robinson, R, Walker, W, Gurll, N, Hawe, D 1991. Insular carcinoma. A distinct thyroid carcinoma with associated Iodine-131 localization. J Nucl Med 32:1358-1.

23. Caplan, R, Abellera, R, Kisken, W 1994. Hürthle cell neoplasms of the thyroid gland. Reassessment of functional capacity. Thyroid 4:243.

24. Cheung, C, Ezzat, S, Ramyar, L, Freeman, J, Asa, S 2000. Molecular basis of Hürthle cell papillary thyroid carcinoma. J Clin Endocrinol Metab 85:878-882.

25. Revised American Thyroid Association management guidelines for patients with thyroid nodules and differentiated thyroid cancer. 2006 Feb (revised 2009 Nov). NGC:007651
American Thyroid Association - Professional Association.

26. DeGroot LJ, Kaplan EL, McCormick M, Straus FH. Natural history, treatment, and course of papillary thyroid carcinoma. J Clin Endocrinol Metab. 1990, 71:414-24.

27. Samaan, N, Schultz, P, Hickey, R, et al. 1992. The results of various modalities of treatment of well differentiated thyroid carcinoma. A retrospective review of 1599 patients. J Clin Endocrinol Metab 75:714-720

28 Hay, I, Grant, C, Bergstralh, E, Thompson, G, van Heerden, J, Goellner, J 1998. Unilateral total lobectomy. Is it sufficient surgical treatment for patients with AMES low-risk papillary thyroid carcinoma? Surgery 124:958-966.

29. Rustad, W, Lindsay, S, Dailey, M 1963. Comparison of the incidence of complications following total and subtotal thyroidectomy for thyroid carcinoma. Surg Gynecol Obstet 116:109.

30. Thompson, N, Harness, J; 1970. Complications of total thyroidectomy for carcinoma. Surg Gynecol Obstet 131:861.

31. Tollefson, H, DeCosse, J 1964. Papillary carcinoma of the thyroid. The case for radical neck dissection. Am J Surg 108:547

32. Grogan RH, Kaplan SP, Cao H, Weiss RE, Degroot LJ, Simon CA, Embia OM, Angelos P, Kaplan EL, Schechter RB. A study of recurrence and death from papillary thyroid cancer with 27 years of median follow-up.Surgery. 2013 Dec;154(6):1436-46

33.Tennvall J, Biorklund A, Moller T et al. Is the EORTC prognostic index of thyroid cancer valid in differentiated thyroid Carcinoma? Cancer 57:1405, 1986.

34. Pasieka JL, Zedenius J, Azuer G et al; Addition of nuclear content to the AMES risk-

group classification for papillary thyroid cancer: Surgery 112:1154, 1992.

35. Hay ID, Bergstralh EJ, Goellner JR, et al. Predicting outcome in papillary thyroid carcinoma. Surgery 114: 1050, 1993.

36. Wong RM, Bresee C, Braunstein GD. Comparison with published systems of a new staging system for papillary and follicular thyroid carcinoma.Thyroid. 2013 May;23(5):566-74

37. Tuttle RM, Tala H, Shah J, Leboeuf R, Ghossein R, Gonen M, Brokhin M, Omry G, Fagin JA, Shaha A.2010 Estimating risk of recurrence in differentiated thyroid cancer after total thyroidectomy and radioactive iodine remnant ablation: using response to therapy variables to modify the initial risk estimates predicted by the new American Thyroid Association staging system. Thyroid. 20:1341-9

38. Castagna MG, Maino F, Cipri C, Belardini V, Theodoropoulou A, Cevenini G, Pacini F. 2011. Delayed risk stratification, to include the response to initial treatment (surgery and radioiodine ablation), has better outcome predictivity in differentiated thyroid cancer patients. Eur J Endocrinol. 165:441-6.

39. Cady, B, Sedgwick, C, Meissner, W, Bookwalter, J, Romagosa, V, Werber, J 1976. Changing clinical; pathologic; therapeutic; and survival patterns of differentiated thyroid carcinoma. Ann Surg 184:541.

40. DeGroot, L, Reilly, M 1982. Comparison of 30- and 50-mCi doses of iodine-131 for thyroid ablation. Ann Intern Med 96:51.

41. Roos, D e a 1999. Review of trials assessing low dose radioactive iodine ablation for thyroid remnants in patients with thyroid cancer. International J Rad Oncol Biol Physiol 44:493-495.

42. Tala Jury HP, Castagna MG, Fioravanti C, Cipri C, Brianzoni E, Pacini F. 2010. Lack of association between urinary iodine excretion and successful thyroid ablation in thyroid cancer patients. J Clin Endocrinol Metab.95:230-7.

43. Karam M, Ianoukakis A, Feustel PJ, Cheema A, Postal ES, Cooper JA. Influence of diagnostic and therapeutic doses on thyroid remnant ablation rates. Nucl Med Commun 24:489-95, 2003.

44. Wartofsky, L, Sherman, S, Gopal, J, Schlumberger, M, Hay, I 1998. The use of radioactive iodine in patients with papillary and follicular thyroid cancer. J Clin Endocrinol Metab 83:4195-4203.

45. Carcangiu, M, Bianchi, S, Savino, D, Voynick, I, Rosai, J 1991. Follicular Hürthle cell tumors of the thyroid gland. Cancer 68:1944-1953..

46. Guimaraes V, DeGroot LJ. Moderate hypothyroidism in preparation for whole body 131-I scintiscans and thyroglobulin testing. Thyroid. 1996, 6:69-73

47. Driedger, AA; Kotowycz, N. Two cases of thyroid carcinoma that were not stimulated by recombinant human thyrotropin. J Clin Endocrinol Metab 89 585-590 2004.

48. Sorvillo, F; Mazziotti,G; Carbone, A; Piscopo, M; Rotondi, M; Cioffi, M; Musto, P; Biondi, B; Iorio, S; Amato, G; Carella, C. Recombinant human thyrotropin reduces serum vascular endothelial growth factor levels in patients monitored for thyroid carcinoma even in the absence of thyroid tissue. J Clin Endocrinol Metab 88 4818-4822 2003.

49. Luster M, Lippi F, Jarzab B, Perros P, Lassmann M, Reiners C, Pacini F. rhTSH-aided radioiodine ablation and treatment of differentiated thyroid carcinoma: a

comprehensive review.Endocr Relat Cancer. 2005 Mar;12(1):49-64.

50. Bachelot, A, Cailleux, A F, Klain, M, et al. 2002 Relationship between tumor burden and serum thyroglobulin level in patients with papillary and follicular thyroid carcinoma. Thyroid 12:707-11.

51. Mazzaferri, E, Kloos, R 2002. Is diagnostic Iodine-131 scanning with recombinant human TSH useful in the follow-up of differentiated thyroid cancer after thyroid ablation? J Clin Endocrinol Metab 87:1490-1498.

52. Wartofsky, L 2002. Using baseline and recombinant human TSH-stimulated tg measurements to manage thyroid cancer without diagnostic 131-I scanning. J Clin Endocrinol Metab 87:1486-1489.

53. Wartofsky, L 2002 Management of low-risk well-differentiated thyroid cancer based only on thyroglobulin measurement after recombinant human thyrotropin. Thyroid 12:583-90.

54. Wartofsky L; rhTSH-Stimulated Thyroglobulin Study Group. Management of low-risk well-differentiated thyroid cancer based only on thyroglobulin measurement after recombinant human thyrotropin. Thyroid. 2002, 12:583-90

55. Pacini F, Schlumberger M, Dralle H, Elisei R, Smit JWA, Wiersinga W and the European Thyroid Cancer Taskforce. European consensus for the management of patients with differentiated thyroid carcinoma of the follicular epithelium. Eur J Endocrinol, 154:1-18, 2006.

56. Spencer C, Fatemi S. Thyroglobulin antibody (TgAb) methods - Strengths, pitfalls and clinical utility for monitoring TgAb-positive patients with differentiated thyroid cancer. Best Pract Res Clin Endocrinol Metab. 2013 Oct;27(5):701-12

57. Van Nostrand, D, Atkins, F, Yeganeh, F, Acio, E, Bursaw, R, Wartofsky, L 2002. Dosimetrically determined doses of radioiodine for the treatment of metastatic thyroid carcinoma. Thyroid 12:121-134.

58. O'Connell, M, Flower, M, Hinton, P, Harmer, C, McCready, V 1993. Radiation dose assessment in radioiodine therapy. Dose-response relationships in differentiated thyroid carcinoma using quantitative scanning and PET. Radiotherapy-Oncology 28:16-26.

59. Sun XS, Sun SR, Guevara N, Marcy PY, Peyrottes I, Lassalle S, Lacout A, Sadoul JL, Santini J, Benisvy D, Lepinoy A, Thariat J. Indications of external beam radiation therapy in non-anaplastic thyroid cancer and impact of innovative radiation techniques. Crit Rev Oncol Hematol. 2013 Apr;86(1):52-68

60. Maxon, H, Thomas, S, Hertzberg, V, et al. 1983. Relation between effective radiation dose and outcome of radioiodine therapy for thyroid cancer. N Engl J Med 309:937.

61. Fatourechi, V, Hay, I, Mullan, B, et al. 2000. Are posttherapy radioiodine scans informative and do they influence subsequent therapy of patients with differentiated thyroid cancer? Thyroid 10:573.

62. Pelikan, D, Lion, H, Hermans, J, Goslings, B 1997. The role of radioactive iodine in the treatment of advanced differentiated thyroid carcinoma. Clin Endocrinol 47:713-720.

63. Menzel, C, Grunwald, F, Schomburg, A, et al. 1996. "High-dose" radioiodine therapy in advanced differentiated thyroid carcinoma. J Nucl Med 37:1496-1503.

64. Taylor, T, Specker, B, Robbins, J, et al. 1998. Outcome after treatment of high-risk papillary and non-Hürthle-cell follicular thyroid carcinoma. Ann Intern Med 129:622-627.

65. Pittas, A, Adler, M, Fazzari, M, et al. 2000. Bone metastases from thyroid carcinoma. clinical characteristics and prognostic variables in one hundred forty-six patients. Thyroid 10:261-268.

66. Van Tol, K, Hew, J, Jager, P, Vermey, A, Dullaart, R, Links, T 2000. .Embolization in combination with radioiodine therapy for bone metastases from differentiated thyroid carcinoma. Clin Endocrinol 52:653-659.

67. Meier, C, Braverman, L, Ebner, S, et al. 1994. Diagnostic use of recombinant human thyrotropin in patients with thyroid carcinoma (phase I/II study). J Clin Endocrinol Metab; 78:188-96..

68. Hamburger, J, Desai, P Mannitol augmentation of I131 uptake in the treatment of thyroid carcinoma. Metabolism 15 1055: 1966.

69 Hamburger, J 1969. Diuretic augmentation of 131-I uptake in inoperable thyroid cancer. N Engl J Med 280:1091.

70. Haq MS, MacCready RV, Harmer CL. Treatment of advanced differentiated thyroid carcinoma with high activity radioiodine therapy. Nucl Med Commun 25:799-805, 2004.

71. Dorn R, Kopp J, Vogt H, Heidenreich P, Carroll RG, Gulec SA.Dosimetry-guided radioactive iodine treatment in patients with metastatic differentiated thyroid cancer: largest safe dose using a risk-adapted approach. J Nucl Med 44:4516, 2003.

72. Pacini, F, Lippi, F, Formica, N, et al. 1987. Therapeutic doses of iodine-131 reveal undiagnosed metastases in thyroid cancer patients with detectable serum thyroglobulin levels. J Nucl Med 28:1888.

73. Koh J-M, Kim ES, Ryu JS, Hong SJ, Kim WB, Shong YK. Effects of therapeutic doses of 131-I in thyroid papillary carcinoma patients with elevated thyroglobulin level and negative 131-I whole-body scan: comparative study. Clin Endocrinol 58:421-427, 2003.

74. Schlumberger, M, Arcangioli, O, Piekarski, J, Tubiana, M, Parmentier, C 1988. Detection and treatment of lung metastases of differentiated thyroid carcinoma in patients with normal chest X-rays. J Nucl Med 29:1790-1794.

75. Pineda, J, Lee, T, Ain, K, Reynolds, J, Robbins, J 1995. Iodine-131 therapy for thyroid cancer patients with elevated thyroglobulin and negative diagnostic scan. J Clin Endocrinol Metab 80:1488.

76. McDougall, I 1997 131-I treatment of 131-I negative whole body scan; and positive thyroglobulin in differentiated thyroid carcinoma. what is being treated? Thyroid 7:669.

77. Fatourechi, V, Hay, I D, Javedan, H, Wiseman, G A, Mullan, B P, Gorman, C A 2002 Lack of impact of radioiodine therapy in tg-positive, diagnostic whole-body scan-negative patients with follicular cell-derived thyroid cancer. J Clin Endocrinol Metab 87:1521-6.

78. Grigsby, P, Siegel, B, Baker, S, Eichling, J 2000. Radiation exposure from outpatient radioactive iodine (131-I) therapy for thyroid carcinoma. J Amer Med Assn 283:2272-2274.

79. American Thyroid Association Taskforce On Radioiodine Safety, Sisson JC, Freitas J, McDougall IR, Dauer LT, Hurley JR, Brierley JD, Edinboro CH, Rosenthal D, Thomas MJ, Wexler JA, Asamoah E, Avram AM, Milas M, Greenlee C. Radiation safety in the treatment of patients with thyroid diseases by radioiodine 131-I : practice recommendations of the American Thyroid Association. Thyroid. 2011, 21:335-46. Erratum in: Thyroid. 2011, 21:689.

80. Seidlin, S, Yalow, R, Siegel, E 1952. Blood radioiodine concentration and blood radiation dosage during I131 therapy for metastatic thyroid carcinoma. J Clin Endocrinol Metab 12:1197.

81. Mandel SJ, Mandel L. Radioactive iodine and the salivary glands. Thyroid 13:265-271, 2003.

82. Raymond, J, Izembart, M, Marliac, V, et al. 1989. Temporary ovarian failure in thyroid cancer patients after thyroid remnant ablation with radioactive iodine. J Clin Endocrinol Metab 69:186.

83. Ceccarelli, C, Battisti, P, Gasperi, M, et al. 1999. Radiation dose to the testes after 131-I therapy for ablation of postsurgical thyroid remnants in patients with differentiated thyroid cancer. J Nucl Med 40:1716.

84. Pochin, E 1960. Leukemia following radioiodine treatment of thyrotoxicosis. Br Med J 2:1545.

85. Wiseman, J, Hales, I, Joasoo, A 1982. Two cases of lymphoma of the parotid gland following ablative radioiodine therapy for thyroid carcinoma. Clin Endocrinol 17:85.

86. Rall, J, Alpers, J, Lewallen, C, Sonenberg, M, Berman, M, Rawson, R 1957. Radiation pneumonitis and fibrosis. A complication of I131 treatment of pulmonary metastases from cancer of the thyroid. J Clin Endocrinol Metab 17:1263.

87. Trunnell, J, Marinelli, L, Duffy, B J, Hill, R, Peacock, W, Rawson, R 1949. The treatment of metastatic thyroid cancer with radioactive iodine. Credits and debits. J Clin Endocrinol Metab 19:1138.

88. Lin, J, Wang, H, Weng, H, Kao, P 1998. Outcome of pregnancy after radioactive iodine treatment for well differentiated thyroid carcinomas. J Endocrinol Invest 21:662-667.

89. Varma, V, Beierwaltes, W, Nofal, M, Nishiyama, R, Copp, J 1437 Treatment of thyroid cancer. Death rates after surgery and after surgery followed by sodium iodide. I131 JAMA: 214.

90. Marcocci, C, Pacini, F, Elisei, R, et al. 1989. Clinical and biologic behavior of bone metastases from differentiated thyroid carcinoma. Surgery 106:960.

91. Saenger, E, Barrett, C, Passino, J, Seltzer, R, Dooley, W 1964. Experiences with I131 in the management of carcinoma of the thyroid. Radiology 83:892.

92. Harness, J, Thompson, N, Sisson, J, Beierwaltes, W 1974. Differentiated thyroid carcinomas. Treatment of distant metastases. Arch Surg 108:410.

93. Solomon, B, Wartofsky, L, Burman, K 1996. Current trends in the management of well differentiated papillary thyroid carcinoma. J Clin Endocrinol Metab 81:333-339.

94. Shands, W, Gatling, R 1970. Cancer of the thyroid. Review of 109 cases. Ann Surg 171:735.

95. Durante C, Haddy N, Baudin E, Leboulleux S, Hartl D, Travagli JP, Caillou B, Ricard M, Lumbroso JD, De Vathaire F, Schlumberger M. Long-term outcome of 444 patients with distant metastases from papillary and follicular thyroid carcinoma: benefits and limits of radioiodine therapy. J Clin Endocrinol Metab. 2006, 91:2892-9.

96. Schlumberger, M 1998. Papillary and follicular thyroid carcinoma. N Engl J Med 338:.297-306.

97. Sherman, S, Tielens, E, Sostre, S, Wharam, M J, Ladenson, P 1994. Clinical utility of

post-treatment radioiodine scans in the management of patients with thyroid cancer. J Clin Endocrinol Metab 78:629.

98. Cailleux, A, Baudin, E, Travagli, J, Ricard, M, Schlumberger, M 2000. Is diagnostic Iodine-131 scanning useful after total thyroid ablation for differentiated thyroid cancer? J Clin Endocrinol Metab 85:175-178.

99. Capezzone, M, Sculli, M, Agate, L, Ceccarelli, C, Pacini, F 2000. Diagnostic 131-I whole body scan after total thyroidectomy and thyroid ablation is useless in thyroid cancer patients with undetectable serum thyroglobulin off l-thyroxine therapy. J Endocrinol Invest (Suppl) 23:3.

100. 515. Charles, M, Dodson, L, Waldeck, N, et al. 1980. Serum thyroglobulin levels predict total body iodine scan findings in patients with treated well-differentiated thyroid carcinoma. Am J Med 69:401.

101. Pacini, F, Pinchera, A, Giani, C, Grasso, L, Baschieri, L 1980. Serum thyroglobulin concentrations and 131-I whole body scans in the diagnosis of metastases from differentiated thyroid carcinoma (after thyroidectomy). Clin Endocrinol 13:107.

102. Barsano, C, Skosey, C, DeGroot, L, Refetoff, S 1982. Serum thyroglobulin in the management of patients with thyroid cancer. Arch Intern Med 142:763.

103. Pacini, F, Pinchera, A, Giani, C, Grasso, L, Doveri, F, Baschieri, L 1980. Serum thyroglobulin in thyroid carcinoma and other thyroid disorders. J Endocrinol Invest 3:283.

104. Johansen, K, Woodhouse, N 1992. Comparison of thyroglobulin and radioiodine scintigraphy during follow-up of patients with differentiated thyroid carcinoma. Eur J Med 1:403-406.

105. Haugen, B, Pacini, F, Reiners, C, et al. 1999. A comparison of recombinant human thyrotropin and thyroid hormone withdrawal for the detection of thyroid remnant or cancer. J Clin Endocrinol Metab 84:3877-3885

106. Fugazzola, L, Mihalich, A, Persani, L, et al. 2002 Highly sensitive serum thyroglobulin and circulating thyroglobulin mRNA evaluations in the management of patients with differentiated thyroid cancer in apparent remission. J Clin Endocrinol Metab 87:3201-8.

107. Elisei R, Vivaldi A, Agate L, Molinaro E, Nencetti C, Grasso L, Pinchera A, Pacini F. Low specificity of blood thyroglobulin messenger ribonucleic acid assay prevents its use in the follow-up of differentiated thyroid cancer patients. J Clin Endocrinol Metab 89:33-9, 2004.

108. Pujol, P, Daures, J-P, Nsakala, N, Baldet, L, Bringer, J, Jaffiol, C 1996. Degree of thyrotropin suppression as a prognostic determinant in differentiated thyroid cancer. J Clin Endocrinol Metab 81:4318-4323.

109. Cooper, D, Specker, B, Ho, M, et al. Thyrotropin suppression and disease progression in patients with differentiated thyroid cancer: results from the National Thyroid Cancer Treatment Cooperative Registry. 1998 Thyroid 8: 737.

110. Marcocci, C, Golia, F, Bruno-Bossio, G, Vignali, E, Pinchera, A 1994. Carefully monitored lecothyroxine suppressive therapy is not associated with bone loss in premenopausal women. . J Clin Endocrinol Metab 78:818-23.

S2-DEFINING RAI REFRACTORY THYROID CANCER: WHEN IS RAI THERAPY UNLIKELY TO ACHIEVE A THERAPEUTIC RESPONSE?

R Michael Tuttle, MD and Mona M. Sabra, MD
Endocrinology Service, Memorial Sloan-Kettering Cancer Center, New York, New York, 10021

INTRODUCTION

For more than 50 years, radioactive iodine has been effectively used to treat metastatic thyroid cancer (1). Dramatic therapeutic responses are often seen when the metastatic foci demonstrate high level avidity for radioactive iodine. These dramatic responses are most common in younger patients with well-differentiated papillary thyroid cancer, in whom radioactive iodine therapy produces dramatic shrinkage of structural disease and results in long-term remission's and excellent survival (2). However, radioactive iodine is often much less effective in older patients who often have a larger volume of disease burden and more poorly differentiated tumors that often concentrate radioactive iodine inefficiently. Furthermore, repeated radioactive iodine administrations are often associated with declining therapeutic effectiveness presumably because of a selection for the non-RAI avid components of the tumor to be the persistent disease (2).

Unfortunately, it is often difficult to determine whether or not metastatic thyroid cancer lesions are likely to be responsive to radioactive iodine therapy since significant therapeutic benefit is occasionally seen even in patients with poorly differentiated thyroid cancer, Hürthle cell carcinoma, widely metastatic follicular thyroid carcinoma and occasionally in patients with large volume metastatic foci. Furthermore, the determination of whether or not radioactive iodine has been an effective therapy for an individual patient is also hampered by the observation that metastatic thyroid cancer can progress very slowly over many years and that serum thyroglobulin may continue to decline for years after initial therapy (3, 4).

These clinical conundrums have led to a pattern of multiple, repeated administrations of radioactive iodine over the years that may or may not have been beneficial. More recently, an increased appreciation of the potential side effects of large cumulative doses of radioactive iodine has led to a reevaluation of the therapeutic benefit of radioactive iodine therapy (5). In addition, the recent availability of potentially effective systemic therapies for non-RAI avid metastatic thyroid cancer has led to a wide range of potential new treatment options for these patients (6). As these systemic therapies become increasingly available, it is critically important to determine when therapeutic administration of radioactive iodine is no longer likely to be effective so that these patients can be offered these novel therapies either as part of clinical trials or as standard of care therapy as these agents gain FDA approval.

Ideally, a direct measurement of the RAI dose achieved within each metastatic lesion in every thyroid cancer patient would allow clinicians to confidently determine whether RAI is likely to be tumoricidal (7-9). Unfortunately, lesional dosimetry is not commonly available in clinical practice making it necessary to use a variety of indirect methods to determine if radioactive iodine therapy has been, or is likely to be, effective in the management of individual patients.

In this review, we will review direct and indirect methods that can be used either in clinical practice or in research studies to determine the RAI avidity of metastatic thyroid cancer. Following that review, we will propose criteria that can be used in routine clinical practice to define RAI refractory disease so that patients with non-RAI avid metastatic disease can avoid excess radioactive iodine administrations that are unlikely to be effective while also minimizing the clinically significant side effects that are associated with large cumulative doses of radioactive iodine.

FACTORS ASSOCIATED WITH SUBOPTIMAL RAI AVIDITY IN METASTATIC THYROID CANCER

As outlined in Figure 1, a wide variety of factors have been shown to be associated with suboptimal RAI avidity in metastatic thyroid cancer. While some of these individual factors may not absolutely define a patient as "RAI refractory", they do provide important clinical clues as to whether or not additional RAI therapy is likely to have a clinical benefit. Assessment of the RAI avidity of metastatic thyroid cancer can be classified based on direct measurements of lesional dosimetry, indirect predictors of RAI avidity, and/or clinical response to previous RAI therapy.

Figure 1

Factors Associated with Suboptimal RAI Avidity in Metastatic Thyroid Cancer
Direct measurement of lesional dosimetry
- Therapeutic RAI predicted to deliver individual lesional dose of < 8,000 cGy

Indirect predictors of RAI avidity
- Negative post-therapy RAI scan
  - Following a properly performed administration of > 30 mCi 131I
  - With either thyroid hormone withdrawal or recombinant human TSH
- Negative diagnostic RAI scan in the setting of structurally identifiable disease
- Markedly positive 18 FDG PET imaging
- Cumulative RAI administered activities > 500-600 mCi

Response to previous RAI therapy
- Structural disease progression 6-12 months after previous RAI therapy
- Rising serum thyroglobulin 6-12 months after previous RAI therapy

USING LESIONAL DOSIMETRY TO ASSESS RAI AVIDITY
Direct measurement of lesional dose

From a clinical perspective, knowledge of the absorbed dose of radiation to individual metastatic lesions would allow more precise predictions with regard to whether or not radioactive iodine therapy would be expected to be clinically effective. Early studies by Maxon et al demonstrated that lesional absorbed doses of 8000-10,000 cGy (rads) were required to reliably achieve tumoricidal activity (8).

In routine clinical practice, assessment of lesional dosimetry can be done by measuring collimated uptake in selected regions of interest (metastatic foci) which are identified by diagnostic whole body scanning (10). Typically several measurements of the region of interest (and appropriate standard for calibration) are made at discrete time points over time 48-72 hours. When integrated with a careful tumor volume measurement (typically by CT scan), reliable estimates of the concentration of RAI achieved within the metastatic foci can be obtained.

More recently, lesional dosimetry utilizing iodine 124 PET imaging has been the subject of investigation, and if clinically validated, is likely to enter clinical practice in the next few years (9, 11, 12). In this approach, a positron emitting form of radioactive iodine (124 iodine) can be used both for diagnostic imaging but also for determination of the concentration of radioactive iodine within individual lesions using standard PET equipment (See Figure 2). Since 124 iodine is commercially available and standard PET imaging equipment can be used for data acquisition and analysis, assimilation of this technique into clinical practice is likely to be relatively easy once the validation studies are complete and 124 iodine is approved for this indication by the FDA.

Figure 2

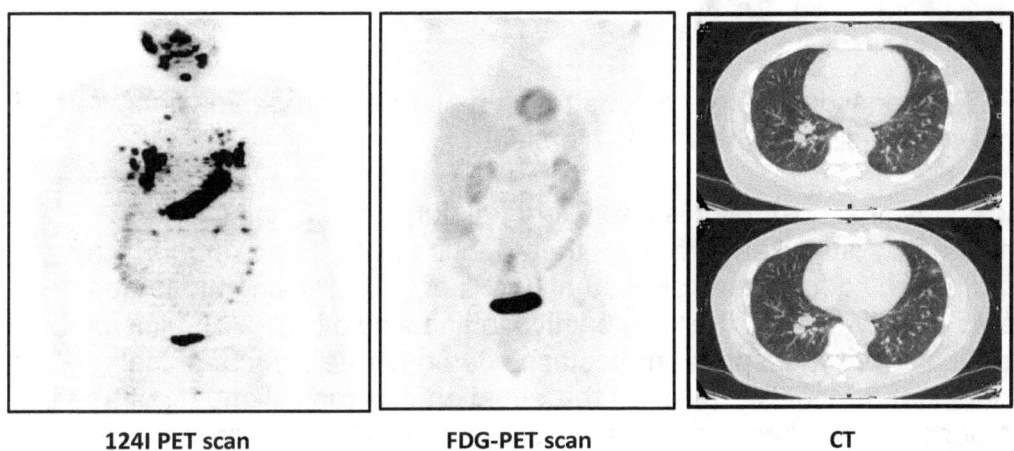

124I PET scan   **FDG-PET scan**   **CT**

Figure 2. Examples of 124 PET imaging (left panel), FDG PET scan (middle panel) and chest CT (right panel) in a patient with metastatic papillary thyroid cancer

Unfortunately, even when the lesional dose is known for each metastatic foci, clinical decision-making is still complex. Individual patients often demonstrate a wide range of absorbed doses across their metastatic lesions (See Figure 3). Furthermore, heterogeneous dose distributions are often seen within large metastatic lesions (12). Conversely, lesional dosimetry cannot be accurately measured in very small lesions. Additionally, lesional dosimetry estimates can change over time and are therefore required with each subsequent consideration of radioactive iodine therapy (13, 14). Therefore, even if lesional dosimetry is performed, clinical decision-making is still required to determine whether or not additional radioactive iodine therapy is likely to be effective.

Heterogeneity in absorbed dose distribution in individual patient

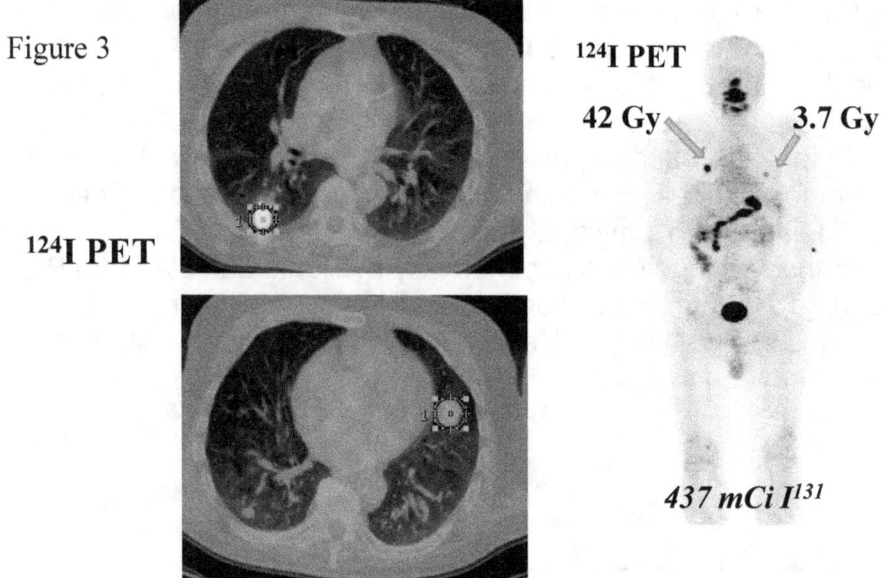

Figure 3. 124 PET lesional dosimetry demonstrating marked heterogeneity in absorbed dose between individual lesions within a single patient.

Nonetheless, lesional dosimetry is often very helpful in determining when radioactive iodine therapy is unlikely to have a therapeutic effect. For example, if all metastatic foci are predicted to receive sub-lethal doses of RAI following the largest safely administered activity of 131I, then radioactive iodine would not be administered. The majority of patients with widespread metastases demonstrate some foci that are very RAI avid and others that are not RAI avid. In this situation, the clinical impact of treating the RAI avid component of the tumor must be assessed clinically. If there is a clinical benefit to treating the RAI avid component of the metastatic disease, then it is reasonable to proceed with additional radioactive iodine therapy. However, if the patient has structurally progressive non-RAI avid metastatic foci, it is possible to classify the patient as having RAI refractory disease for purposes of clinical trials even if clinically insignificant small foci of disease retain RAI avidity.

Indirect correlates of lesional dose

While direct measurements of lesional dosimetry have the potential to provide objective data that can be used to guide treatment decisions, they are not available for the majority of thyroid cancer patients. In clinical practice, radionuclide scanning is often used to provide information about whether or not metastatic lesions are likely to respond to radioactive iodine. The most widely accepted clinical definition of RAI refractory requires demonstration of the lack of radioactive iodine uptake within metastatic lesions on a properly done radioactive iodine post therapy scan obtained after administration of therapeutic doses of radioactive iodine (greater than 30 mCi). While there is some data to indicate that lesional dosimetry can be somewhat higher following thyroid hormone withdrawal preparation than with recombinant human TSH administration in some patients, we accept a negative post therapy scan after recombinant human TSH stimulated radioactive iodine therapy as adequate evidence that the metastatic foci are RAI refractory. The lack of visualization of the metastatic foci after high dose radioactive iodine therapy is certainly a valid and reliable indicator of poor lesional dosimetry.

More recently, Sabra et al demonstrated a lack of therapeutic effectiveness of radioactive iodine in clinical scenarios were structurally identifiable disease was associated with a negative diagnostic whole body scan even when the post therapy scan demonstrated some degree of RAI avidity (15). In our view, the inability to visualize radioactive iodine uptake within structurally significant metastatic foci on the diagnostic 2mCi radioactive iodine scan is in indirect indicator of low absorbed dose. In this situation, even though the metastatic foci can be visualized after high dose therapy, it is quite unlikely that a tumoricidal dose can be achieved since the lesion concentrated radioactive iodine so poorly that it could not be visualized on diagnostic scanning. Internal unpublished data does show that these patients have very low lesional dosimetry when evaluated on 124 iodine PET imaging (See Figure 4).

Figure 4

**64 year old
Stage IV, Follicular Thyroid Cancer**

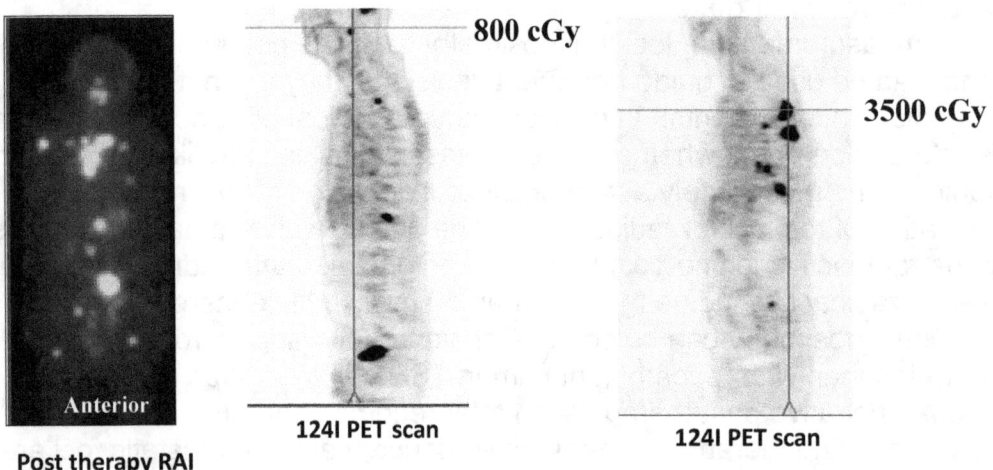

Figure 4. Example of a post therapy RAI scan showing multiple RAI avid skeletal metastases in which lesional dosimetry predicts subtherapeutic doses of RAI (corresponding diagnostic RAI scan was negative).

18 FDG PET scanning can also be used as a predictor of therapeutic effectiveness of radioactive iodine (16). We have previously demonstrated that even high dose radioactive iodine therapy (430 ± 243 mCi cumulative dose) did not decrease the FDG tumor volume, subsequent SUV, or serum thyroglobulin in a cohort of 25 differentiated thyroid cancer with FDG avid metastases (mean maximum SUV 9.3 ± 1, range 2.3-30) (16). In addition, FDG positivity correlates with structural disease progression and mortality (17). Therefore, we consider patient's that have metastatic foci which have significant FDG avidity (arbitrarily defined as an SUV > 5-10), to have disease that is likely to be radioactive iodine resistant, and to progress. We then move on to consideration for novel therapies rather than repeated administrations of radioactive iodine. Conversely, low level FDG avidity (SUV < 2) does not preclude the possibility that the lesion could be RAI avid and potentially could be responsive to additional RAI therapy.

While the specific histology generally correlates with RAI avidity, none have sufficient sensitivity or specificity to determine whether or not radioactive iodine is likely to be effective therapy. For example, we have seen significant uptake of radioactive iodine in perhaps 10-20% of our patients with either Hürthle cell carcinoma or poorly differentiated phenotypes. Similarly, older patients, particularly with follicular thyroid cancers, often demonstrate the clinical benefit from radioactive iodine therapy. Conversely, it is not uncommon to see metastatic lesions from a classic papillary thyroid carcinoma fail to concentrate significant amounts of radioactive iodine.   Therefore, we do not use tumor histology or patient age as primary indicators to define RAI refractory disease.

Similarly, while the molecular profile of radioactive iodine avid metastatic disease differs from that of RAI refractory disease, the molecular profile does not adequately predict a therapeutic response (18, 19). Radioactive iodine refractory disease is enriched in BRAF mutations which have been shown in pre-clinical and clinical models to down regulate the sodium iodine symporter rendering radioactive iodine therapy less effective (20, 21). Even though the significantly higher prevalence of RAS mutations present in RAI avid disease correlates with the likelihood of visualizing metastatic disease on diagnostic RAI scans, the structural response to therapy was not significantly different across the mutational profiles of patient's with RAI avid distant metastases (19).

Large cumulative administered activities of radioactive iodine can also serve as a clinical indicator that additional radioactive iodine therapy is unlikely to be effective. Clinically significant therapeutic effects are very rare in patients that have received a cumulative administered activity of 600 mCi or more (2). Therefore, in the absence of a well documented clinical benefit following the last administered activity of radioactive iodine, it is unlikely that a significant additional therapeutic effect will be seen with cumulative activities exceeding 500-600 mCi.

USING CLINICAL RESPONSE TO PREVIOUS RAI TREATMENTS TO ASSESS RAI AVIDITY

Since it is unusual for a single administration of radioactive iodine to induce remission in patients with metastatic disease, we usually have the benefit of evaluating the effectiveness of the previous radioactive iodine dose when determining whether additional treatments may be helpful. From a clinical perspective, structural disease progression within 6-12 months after a properly administered dose of radioactive iodine would serve as the best evidence that the patient has RAI refractory disease. Once again, it is important to emphasize, that structural disease progression after properly administered RAI therapy constitutes one of the main definitions of RAI refractory disease even if the diagnostic or post therapy scan obtained with the previous treatment was positive. As we have described, planar scanning can identify metastatic lesions even when metastatic foci receive sub-lethal doses of radioactive iodine.

Quite often, the best clinical response to RAI therapy is stable disease. It is usually difficult to determine if the RAI therapy contributed to disease stability, or whether the natural history of an individual patient's disease was destined to be stable/very slow growth even without additional RAI therapy. Therefore, a failure of metastatic lesions to decrease in size after a therapeutic dose does not necessarily mean that RAI therapy was ineffective.

It is worth emphasizing that classification of a patient as radioactive iodine refractory on the basis of response to previous treatments requires a knowledge that the previous treatments were done correctly. We have seen several instances of patients classified as being unresponsive to radioactive iodine who were consistently iodine contaminated with contrast agents in the days preceding their radioactive iodine therapies. While the details of previous therapies are often not available, it is worthwhile reviewing with the patient their potential exposure to excess iodine either through the diet or medical imaging, their method of preparation for radioactive iodine therapy, and the timing of the imaging following radioactive iodine therapy.

While serum thyroglobulin is one of the key components to response to therapy assessments, recent data demonstrates that serum thyroglobulin values may continue to fall for years after initial therapy (3, 4). This is been demonstrated both following radioactive iodine remnant ablation (22), and subsequent to therapeutic doses of radioactive iodine in pediatric thyroid cancer (3). Therefore, rising thyroglobulin values 6-12 months after a therapeutic dose of radioactive iodine would provide biochemical evidence that the previous administered activity of RAI was suboptimally effective.

PRACTICAL CLINICAL DECISION MAKING: DEFINING RAI REFRACTORY DISEASE
In the ideal world, direct measurements utilizing either collimated uptake in selected regions of interest or 124 PET technology would be used to define RAI refractory disease as metastatic foci that would achieve a lesional dose < 8,000 rads after therapeutic administration of RAI.

However, since lesional dosimetry is usually not available in most clinical situations, the definition of RAI refractory disease in most patients will rely on documentation of:
1. A negative post-therapy RAI scan after a properly administered RAI therapy
2. Structural disease progression within 6-12 months of a properly administered RAI therapy
   or
3. Rising serum thyroglobulin within 6-12 months after a properly administered RAI therapy

Furthermore, while not definitively classifying a patient as being completely refractory to RAI, the following clinical factors make it much less likely that RAI therapy will achieve a clinically significant therapeutic response:
1. A negative diagnostic whole body RAI scan in the setting of structurally identifiable disease
2. A positive FDG PET scan with an SUV > 5-10
3. Cumulative administered activities of > 500-600 mCi RAI.

CONCLUSIONS
In the future, we are hopeful that more widespread use of lesional dosimetry will lead to better decision making with regard to be able to objectively define RAI refractory disease. Until then, it will be necessary to continue to define RAI refractory disease on the basis of indirect predictors of RAI avidity and clinical assessments of the effectiveness of previous RAI therapies.

References

1. Lee SL 2012 Radioactive iodine therapy. Curr Opin Endocrinol Diabetes Obes **19**:420-8.
2. Durante C, Haddy N, Baudin E, Leboulleux S, Hartl D, Travagli JP, Caillou B, Ricard M, Lumbroso JD, De Vathaire F, Schlumberger M 2006 Long-term outcome of 444 patients with distant metastases from papillary and follicular thyroid carcinoma: benefits and limits of radioiodine therapy. J Clin Endocrinol Metab **91**:2892-9.
3. Biko J, Reiners C, Kreissl MC, Verburg FA, Demidchik Y, Drozd V 2011 Favourable course of disease after incomplete remission on (131)I therapy in children with pulmonary metastases of papillary thyroid carcinoma: 10 years follow-up. Eur J Nucl Med Mol Imaging **38**:651-5.
4. Durante C, Montesano T, Attard M, Torlontano M, Monzani F, Costante G, Meringolo D, Ferdeghini M, Tumino S, Lamartina L, Paciaroni A, Massa M, Giacomelli L, Ronga G, Filetti S 2012 Long-term surveillance of papillary thyroid cancer patients who do not undergo postoperative radioiodine remnant ablation: is there a role for serum thyroglobulin measurement? J Clin Endocrinol Metab **97**:2748-53.
5. Lee SL 2010 Complications of radioactive iodine treatment of thyroid carcinoma. J Natl Compr Canc Netw **8**:1277-86; quiz 1287.
6. Haugen BR, Sherman SI 2013 Evolving approaches to patients with advanced differentiated thyroid cancer. Endocr Rev **34**:439-55.
7. Lassmann M, Reiners C, Luster M 2010 Dosimetry and thyroid cancer: the individual dosage of radioiodine. Endocr Relat Cancer **17**:R161-72.
8. Maxon HR, Thomas SR, Hertzberg VS, Kereiakes JG, Chen IW, Sperling MI, Saenger EL 1983 Relation between effective radiation dose and outcome of radioiodine therapy for thyroid cancer. N Engl J Med **309**:937-41.
9. Pentlow KS, Graham MC, Lambrecht RM, Daghighian F, Bacharach SL, Bendriem B, Finn RD, Jordan K, Kalaigian H, Karp JS, Robeson WR, Larson SM 1996 Quantitative imaging of iodine-124 with PET. J Nucl Med **37**:1557-62.
10. Siegel JA, Thomas SR, Stubbs JB, Stabin MG, Hays MT, Koral KF, Robertson JS, Howell RW, Wessels BW, Fisher DR, Weber DA, Brill AB 1999 MIRD pamphlet no. 16: Techniques for quantitative radiopharmaceutical biodistribution data acquisition and analysis for use in human radiation dose estimates. J Nucl Med **40**:37S-61S.
11. Freudenberg LS, Jentzen W, Petrich T, Fromke C, Marlowe RJ, Heusner T, Brandau W, Knapp WH, Bockisch A 2010 Lesion dose in differentiated thyroid carcinoma metastases after rhTSH or thyroid hormone withdrawal: 124I PET/CT dosimetric comparisons. Eur J Nucl Med Mol Imaging **37**:2267-76.
12. Sgouros G, Kolbert KS, Sheikh A, Pentlow KS, Mun EF, Barth A, Robbins RJ, Larson SM 2004 Patient-specific dosimetry for 131I thyroid cancer therapy using 124I PET and 3-dimensional-internal dosimetry (3D-ID) software. J Nucl Med **45**:1366-72.
13. Chiesa C, Castellani MR, Vellani C, Orunesu E, Negri A, Azzeroni R, Botta F, Maccauro M, Aliberti G, Seregni E, Lassmann M, Bombardieri E 2009

Individualized dosimetry in the management of metastatic differentiated thyroid cancer. Q J Nucl Med Mol Imaging **53**:546-61.

14. Samuel AM, Rajashekharrao B, Shah DH 1998 Pulmonary metastases in children and adolescents with well-differentiated thyroid cancer. J Nucl Med **39**:1531-6.

15. Sabra MM, Grewal RK, Tala H, Larson SM, Tuttle RM 2012 Clinical outcomes following empiric radioiodine therapy in patients with structurally identifiable metastatic follicular cell-derived thyroid carcinoma with negative diagnostic but positive post-therapy 131I whole-body scans. Thyroid **22**:877-83.

16. Wang W, Larson SM, Tuttle RM, Kalaigian H, Kolbert K, Sonenberg M, Robbins RJ 2001 Resistance of [18f]-fluorodeoxyglucose-avid metastatic thyroid cancer lesions to treatment with high-dose radioactive iodine. Thyroid **11**:1169-75.

17. Robbins RJ, Wan Q, Grewal RK, Reibke R, Gonen M, Strauss HW, Tuttle RM, Drucker W, Larson SM 2006 Real-time prognosis for metastatic thyroid carcinoma based on 2-[18F]fluoro-2-deoxy-D-glucose-positron emission tomography scanning. J Clin Endocrinol Metab **91**:498-505.

18. Ricarte-Filho J, Ganly I, Rivera M, Katabi N, Fu W, Shaha A, Tuttle RM, Fagin JA, Ghossein R 2012 Papillary thyroid carcinomas with cervical lymph node metastases can be stratified into clinically relevant prognostic categories using oncogenic BRAF, the number of nodal metastases, and extra-nodal extension. Thyroid **22**:575-84.

19. Sabra MM, Dominguez JM, Grewal RK, Larson SM, Ghossein RA, Tuttle RM, Fagin JA 2013 Clinical outcomes and molecular profile of differentiated thyroid cancers with radioiodine-avid distant metastases. J Clin Endocrinol Metab **98**:E829-36.

20. Riesco-Eizaguirre G, Gutierrez-Martinez P, Garcia-Cabezas MA, Nistal M, Santisteban P 2006 The oncogene BRAF V600E is associated with a high risk of recurrence and less differentiated papillary thyroid carcinoma due to the impairment of Na+/I- targeting to the membrane. Endocr Relat Cancer **13**:257-69.

21. Xing M, Westra WH, Tufano RP, Cohen Y, Rosenbaum E, Rhoden KJ, Carson KA, Vasko V, Larin A, Tallini G, Tolaney S, Holt EH, Hui P, Umbricht CB, Basaria S, Ewertz M, Tufaro AP, Califano JA, Ringel MD, Zeiger MA, Sidransky D, Ladenson PW 2005 BRAF mutation predicts a poorer clinical prognosis for papillary thyroid cancer. J Clin Endocrinol Metab **90**:6373-9.

22. Padovani RP, Robenshtok E, Brokhin M, Tuttle RM 2012 Even without additional therapy, serum thyroglobulin concentrations often decline for years after total thyroidectomy and radioactive remnant ablation in patients with differentiated thyroid cancer. Thyroid **22**:778-83.

S3-SELECTION OF PATIENTS FOR TKI TREATMENT

Furio Pacini, MD Professor of Endocrinology, Director, Section of Endocrinology and Metabolism
University of Siena, Siena, Italy

Martin Schlumberger , MD Professor of Oncology, University of Paris-Sud, Director, Nuclear Medicine and Endocrine Tumors Division, Institut Gustave-Roussy, Villejuif, Paris, France.

Patients with advanced DTC who are refractory to ^{131}I treatment have a life expectancy of 3-6 years and represent a group for whom there is a clear unmet medical need (1). Radioiodine refractory thyroid cancer is not common, with an estimated incidence of four cases per million population year (5% of patients with clinical thyroid cancer, 250 patients per year in France) (2,3). It occurs more frequently in older patients, in those with large metastases or with poorly differentiated thyroid cancer, and in those with high FDG uptake on PET scan (1, 4).

This review proposes a definition for refractory thyroid cancer, and defines those patients who are candidates for treatment with TKIs.

DEFINITION OF REFRACTORY THYROID CANCER

In all patients treated with ^{131}I, treatment efficacy is assessed by functional parameters (serum Tg level during l-thyroxine therapy and following hormone withdrawal or rhTSH injections, and quantitative ^{131}I uptake in metastases on post-therapy WBS) and also by anatomical imaging with CT scan and MRI. Favorable responses are characterized by parallel decreases in tumor volume on anatomical imaging, ^{131}I uptake, and serum Tg levels. In contrast, a decrease in ^{131}I uptake without a decrease in tumor volume denotes the destruction of differentiated cells with high uptake and the persistence of poorly differentiated foci that will progress. These patients should then be considered DTC refractory to ^{131}I treatment, and they fall into six categories:

a) *Patients with metastatic disease that does not take-up* [131]I *at the time of initial treatment.* For these patients there is evidence that treatment with ^{131}I does not provide any benefit. This group includes patients with structurally evident disease with no ^{131}I uptake on a diagnostic whole-body scan (WBS), because in such patients uptake when present on post-therapy scans will not be sufficient to induce benefit (5).

b) *Patients whose tumors lose the ability to take-up* [131]I *after previous evidence of uptake.* This is due to the eradication by ^{131}I treatment of differentiated cells able to take-up ^{131}I but not of poorly differentiated cells that do not take-up [131]I. Progression is likely to occur in these poorly differentiated cells

c) *Patients with* [131]I *uptake retained in some lesions but not in others.* This is frequently seen in patients with multiple large metastases as shown by [124]I studies on PET scan (6) and by comparing results of imaging modalities (FDG-PET or diagnostic CT scans) with ^{131}I WBS. In such patients, progression is likely to occur in metastases without ^{131}I uptake (in particular when FDG uptake is present) and ^{131}I treatment will not be beneficial (4, 7,

8)

d) *Patients with metastatic disease that progresses despite significant uptake of [131]I*. It has been clearly shown that if progression occurs following a course of adequate radioiodine treatment, subsequent ^{131}I treatment will be ineffective (9).

e) *Less clear is the situation for patients with persistent visible ^{131}I uptake in all residual lesions who are not cured despite several treatment courses but whose disease does not progress according to RECIST criteria.* For these patients, the probability of obtaining a cure with further ^{131}I treatment is low (1) and side effects may significantly increase, including the risk of secondary cancers and leukemias (10). It is controversial as to whether these patients (particularly after receiving more than 600 mCi of ^{131}I) should be considered ^{131}I-refractory and whether ^{131}I treatment should be abandoned. The decision to continue ^{131}I treatment in such patients is generally based on their response to previous treatment courses, persistence of a significant level of ^{131}I uptake on the previous post-therapy WBS, low FDG uptake in tumor foci, and absence of side effects.

f) *Finally, there is a subgroup of patients with advanced disease for whom thyroidectomy is not feasible.* In such patients, ^{131}I treatment is usually not administered because ^{131}I is ineffective when the thyroid gland is still present and ^{131}I uptake status cannot be assessed. These patients could be managed as iodine-refractory patients, or if desired, treated with RAI to destroy the thyroid..

TREATMENT OF REFRACTORY THYROID CANCER--ACTIVE SURVEILLANCE (Table 1)

Once ^{131}I treatment is terminated, L-thyroxine treatment is maintained to suppress TSH secretion and focal treatment of metastases is performed whenever needed. This may include surgery, external radiation beam therapy, and thermo-ablation (radiofrequency or cryo-ablation and cement injection). Also, because bone metastases may induce skeletal related events at short term interval (11), bisphosphonate or denosumab treatment may be effective in patients with bone metastases.

Active surveillance includes a FDG-PET/CT scan or a CT scan of the neck, chest, abdomen and pelvis with contrast, at an interval that is dictated by the pace of prior disease-progression if known, and typically a period of at least one year. Most patients with refractory advanced disease have an aggressive course and a life expectancy of 3-6 years after the discovery of distant metastases. However, metastatic DTC can be asymptomatically stable for long periods of time, in particular in young patients with small lung metastases from a well differentiated papillary or follicular carcinoma and in such patients the benefits of novel therapies may be largely outweighed by drug toxicities.

Table 1--MANAGEMENT OF REFRACTORY DTC
L-T4 treatment with serum TSH <0.1mU/l
Focal treatments when needed
Imaging follow-up every 4-6 months
STABLE DISEASE- continued active follow-up
PROGRESSION : >20% BY RECIST criteria in 6-12 months and significant tumor burden
INCLUSION IN A TRIAL- --Chemotherapy-low efficacy, significant toxicity (eg-doxorubicin=<5% PR, median PFS= 7 months) --Targeted Therapy as first line (ATA, Cooper, Thyroid 2009, 19 :1167)

TREATMENT OF REFRACTORY THYROID CANCER--INDICATION FOR SYSTEMIC THERAPY

The decision to initiate systemic treatment is based on several parameters, including tumor burden, disease progression, symptoms, or high risk of local complications.

a) *Progression rate can be evaluated by the doubling time of serum Tg (12)*,

b) *Progression should always be confirmed before initiating a treatment with TKI by imaging using Response Evaluation Criteria in Solid Tumor (RECIST) (13).* RECIST consists in measuring the longest diameter of each target lesion (lesion >1cm in diameter) at each imaging control and in comparing the sum of these diameters: progression is defined by an increase of this sum by 20% or by the appearance of new lesions; partial response is defined by a decrease in this sum by 30% and complete response is the disappearance of all visible lesion.

Patients with multiple lesions >1-2 cm and with progression within less than 12 months are considered for systemic treatment. On the contrary, patients with few and/or small lung lesions <1cm, and those with no evidence of progression are considered for active follow-up (2).

c) *Some patients with large tumor burden and lacking ^{131}I uptake and for whom there is no data on progression, may be considered for systemic treatment based on uptake of FDG on PET scanning or even on primary tumor histology (7,8), but only when active surveillance is not feasible, or there is a high risk of complications.*

CHOICE OF SYSTEMIC THERAPY

In the past, cytotoxic chemotherapy was used in these patients, but response rates obtained with doxorubicin, the most frequently used agent ranged from 0% to 20%, all responses being partial and transient, and toxicity was significant. The combination with cisplatinum did not improve the efficacy but increased the toxicity (14). Experience is limited with other cytotoxic agents, but reported results were not better than with doxrubicin, and for this reason the ATA recommendations stated in 2009 that kinase inhibitors should be used as first line treatment in patients with refractory DTC in whom progression has been documented. However, toxicities of kinase inhibitors are significant and include fatigue, diarrhea, hypertension and skin toxicities. They occurred in the majority of patients and led to dose reduction in 11–73% of patients and to drug withdrawal in 7–25%. This is why patients' education is mandatory and why these treatments should be managed by experienced teams.

Also, tumor responses were observed in only a fraction of patients and most were partial and transient; improvement of progression free survival has been documented in only one phase 2 trials (15) and in one phase 3 trial (16). There is no evidence that treatment at an early stage may be more efficient than a treatment performed at a later stage when progression has been documented. The duration of treatment is not yet validated and, for this reason, treatment is usually given as long as toxicities remain manageable and there is no evidence of tumor progression. This is the rationale for initiating these treatments only in patients with significant tumour burden and with documented progressive disease.

References

1. Durante C, Haddy N, Baudin E, Leboulleux S, Hartl D, Travagli JP, Caillou B, Ricard M, Lumbroso JD, De Vathaire F, Schlumberger M. Long-term outcome of 444 patients with distant metastases from papillary and follicular thyroid carcinoma: benefits and limits of radioiodine therapy. *J Clin Endocrinol Metab.* 2006; 91:2892-9

2. Xing MM, Haugen B, Schlumberger M. Progress in molecular-based management of differentiated thyroid cancer. *Lancet* 2013; 381: 1058–698.

3. Schlumberger M, Brose M, Elisei R, Leboulleux S, Luster M, Pitoia F, Pacini F Definition and Management of Radioactive Iodine-Refractory Differentiated Thyroid Cancer: Recommendations by an International Expert Panel. Lancet Endocrinol 2014

4. Robbins RJ, Wan Q, Grewal RK, Reibke R, Gonen M, Strauss HW, Tuttle RM, Drucker W, Larson SM. Real-time prognosis for metastatic thyroid carcinoma based on 2-[18F]fluoro-2-deoxy-D-glucose-positron emission tomography scanning. *J Clin Endocrinol Metab.* 2006; 91:498-505.

5. Sabra MM, Grewal RK, Tala H, Larson SM, Tuttle RM. Clinical outcomes following empiric radioiodine therapy in patients with structurally identifiable metastatic follicular cell-derived thyroid carcinoma with negative diagnostic but positive post-therapy 131I whole-body scans. *Thyroid* 2012; 22: 877-83.

6. Sgouros G, Kolbert KS, Sheikh A, Pentlow KS, Mun EF, Barth A, Robbins RJ, Larson SM. Patient-specific dosimetry for 131I thyroid cancer therapy using 124I PET and 3-dimensional-internal dosimetry (3D-ID) software. *J Nucl Med.* 2004; 45:1366-72.

7. Deandreis D, Al Ghuzlan A, Leboulleux S, Lacroix L, Garsi JP, Talbot M, Lumbroso J, Baudin E, Caillou B, Bidart JM, Schlumberger M. Do histological, immunohistochemical and metabolic (radioiodine and fluorodeoxyglucose uptake) patterns of metastatic thyroid cancer correlate with patient outcome? *Endocr Relat Cancer* 2011; 18:159-69.

8. Rivera M, Ghossein RA, Schoder H, Gomez D, Larson SM, Tuttle RM. Histopathologic characterization of radioactive iodine-refractory fluorodeoxyglucose-positron emission tomography-positive thyroid carcinoma. *Cancer* 2008;113: 48-56.

9. Vaisman F, Tala H, Grewal R, Tuttle RM. In differentiated thyroid cancer, an incomplete structural response to therapy is associated with significantly worse clinical outcomes than only an incomplete thyroglobulin response. *Thyroid* 2011;21:1317-22.

10. Rubino C, De Vathaire F, Dottorini ME, Hall P, Schvartz C, Couette JE, Dondon MG, Abbas MT, Langlois C, Schlumberger M. Second primary malignancies in thyroid cancer patients. *Br J Cancer* 2003; 89: 1638-44.

11. Farooki A, Leung V, Tala H, Tuttle RM. Skeletal-related events due to bone metastases from differentiated thyroid cancer. J Clin Endocrinol Metab. 2012; 97: 2433-9.

12. Miyauchi A, Kudo T, Miya A, Kobayashi K, Ito Y, Takamura Y et al. Prognostic impact of serum thyroglobulin doubling-time under thyrotropin suppression in patients with papillary thyroid carcinoma who underwent total thyroidectomy. Thyroid 2011;21:707-16.

13. Eisenhauer EA, Therasse P, Bogaerts J, Schwartz LH, Sargent D, Ford R, Dancey J, Arbuck S, Gwyther S, Mooney M, Rubinstein L, Shankar L, Dodd L, Kaplan R, Lacombe D, Verweij J. New response evaluation criteria in solid tumours: revised RECIST guideline (version 1.1). Eur J Cancer. 2009;45:228-47

14. Sherman SI. Cytotoxic chemotherapy for differentiated thyroid carcinoma. Clin Oncol (R Coll Radiol) 2010;22: 464-8.

15. Leboulleux S, Bastholt L, Krause T, de la Fouchardiere C, Tennvall J, Awada A et al. Vandetanib in locally advanced or metastatic differentiated thyroid cancer: a randomised, double-blind, phase 2 trial. Lancet Oncol 2012;13: 897-905.

16. Brose MS, Nutting CM, Jarzab B, Elisei R, Siena S, Bastholt L, de la Fouchardiere C, Pacini F, Paschke R, Shong YK, Sherman SI, Smit JWA, Chung J, Kappeler C, Pena C, Molnar I, Schlumberger M Sorafenib in locally advanced or metastatic, radioactive iodine-refractory, differentiated thyroid cancer: a randomized, double-blind, phase 3 trial. ASCO 2013

S4-NEW TREATMENT ALGORITHMS FOR SYSTEMIC THERAPY IN MANAGING AGGRESSIVE THYROID CANCER

Joshua Klopper and Bryan Haugen
University of Colorado School of Medicine

An important subset of patients with well differentiated thyroid cancer (WDTC) will develop progressive local or metastatic disease that no longer responds to the best targeted therapy, radioiodine (RAI). It is important to remember that directed therapy may still be appropriate with patients with widely metastatic disease if only one or a few lesions are progressing or symptomatic but the majority of the disease is stable and asymptomatic. Additionally, with advances in molecular oncology and therapies targeted at oncoproteins, patients with advanced thyroid cancer have more options for therapy than at any other time(1).

For persistent disease in the neck, when surgery is not a viable option, other directed modalities can be considered. External beam radiotherapy to growing regional disease can be considered. Newer modalities include radiofrequency ablation (RFA) and percutaneous ethanol ablation (PEI). Radiofrequency ablation is still primarily used in referral centers and has not been adopted in widespread practice(2). PEI is used more commonly and is useful to treat loco-regional nodes/masses (3). Though the strategy can only be used for a small number of lesions at one time, it is minimally invasive and has rare morbidity(4). However, in the setting of distant, progressive metastases, the utility of targeting an isolated lesion is of questionable value and systemic therapy is likely more appropriate.

TYROSINE KINASE INHIBITOR TREATMENT
In the setting of progressive radioiodine refractory thyroid cancer metastases, the availability of multi-targeted tyrosine kinase inhibitors (TKIs) has allowed beneficial and generally well tolerated therapy. At this point, the only TKI with an FDA approved indication for radioiodine resistant metastatic thyroid cancer is sorafenib (marketed as Nexavar) which received approval in November 2013. However, there are numerous other TKIs approved for medullary thyroid cancer (MTC) as well as other solid tumors that have been studied as well. As has been described in the earlier chapters of this symposium, systemic therapy is appropriate to consider for patients with RAI resistant therapy that is progressive; where a "watch and wait" strategy is no longer acceptable. The verification of progression is important as these therapies tend to provide a tumorostatic response as opposed to a tumorcidal effect as will be shown by the clinical trials data. Even when thyroid cancer is RAI refractory, and occasionally even when positron emission tomography (PET) positive, metastatic disease can be quite stable for some time, even years. In the absence of progression, therefore a drug that does not cause measurable regression of disease is likely to have an unacceptably high side effect to benefit ratio.

TKI therapies target multiple oncoproteins and oncogenic signaling pathways. A detailed explanation of how each TKI targets individual receptors and pathways is beyond the scope of this chapter but has been recently reviewed(5). Briefly, TKIs may inhibit activation of the mitogen-activated protein kinase pathway (MAPK) as well as the PI3K-AKT pathway in tumor cells. Additionally, they can target vascular endothelial growth factor receptor (VEFGFR), endothelial growth factor receptor (EGFR) and mitogen activated protein kinase enzyme (MET) on vascular endothelial cells. Most TKIs target more than one of these pathways/receptors. Table 1 demonstrates some of the targets of the TKIs that have been studied in published reports.

Table 1- Phase II Thyroid cancer clinical trials

Target	RET RET/PTC	EGFR	MET	BRAF	MEK	FLT3	VEFGFR (1-3)	PDGFR	c-kit
Axitinib							X	x	X
Gefitinib		x							
Motesanib	x						X	x	X
Pazopanib							X		
Selumetenib					x				
Sorafenib	x			x			X	x	X
Sunitinib	x					x	X	x	X
Vandetanib	x	x					X		

Targets of TKIs studied in published, peer-reviewed phase II clinical trials for advanced DTC. Adapted from (5;28)

Other TKIs have been studied in advanced DTC and to date have only been presented in abstract form and therefore are not described in detail in this chapter. These include lenvatinib and cabozantinib. As of the writing of this chapter, only one phase III trial of a TKI in advanced DTC has been completed studying sorafenib (the DECISION trial). This trial led to FDA approval of DTC as an indication for use, yet has still only been presented in abstract form (6). Additionally, phase III trials of other TKIs in advanced thyroid cancer are ongoing. A synopsis of phase II trial outcomes is summarized in Table 2 and the trials are briefly described in more detail below.

Axitinib(7) – 60 subjects (30 papillary, 15 follicular, 11 medullary, 2 anaplastic and 2 other) were enrolled in a multicenter single arm open label study of patients with advanced thyroid cancer that were not amenable to surgery or radioiodine. Axitinib was initiated at 5mg orally twice daily BIDand response by RECIST criteria was the primary end point. 30% of patients had a partial response (PR) and 38% had stable disease (SD). Median progression free survival (PFS) was 18 months. Thirteen percent of subjects discontinued the trial drug due to adverse events.

Gefitinib(8) – 27 subjects (11 papillary, 6 follicular, 5 anaplastic, 4 medullary and 1 hürthle cell thyroid cancers) were enrolled in a multicenter single arm open label study of patients with advanced thyroid cancer not amenable to radioiodine therapy. Gefitinib was initiated at 250mg daily (QD) and response by RECIST criteria was the primary endpoint. There were no PR, but at 6 months 24% of subjects had SD. Median PFS was 3.7 months. Two patients discontinued therapy due to toxicity.

Motesanib (9) – 93 subjects (57 papillary, 36 follicular/hürthle cell thyroid cancers) were enrolled in a multi- institution, international open label study of patients with radioiodine resistant DTC. Motesanib 125mg orally (PO) QD was initiated and the primary end point was objective tumor response by RECIST criteria. 14% of patients had a PR and 67% had SD for 24 weeks or longer. Thirteen percent of patients discontinued treatment due to toxicity.

Pazopanib(10) – 37 subjects (15 papillary, 11 follicular, 11 hürthle cell thyroid cancers) were enrolled in a multi-institution open label study of patients with metastatic, progressive, radioiodine refractory DTC. Pazopanib 800mg PO QD was initiated and the primary end point was objective tumor response by RECIST criteria. 49% of patients had a PR. PFS at one year was 47% with a median duration of PFS of 11.7 months. Only one patient requested withdrawal of treatment.

Selumetenib(11) – 20 subjects (5 papillary, 8 tall-cell variant papillary, 7 poorly differentiated thyroid cancers) were enrolled in a single-institution open label study of patients with radioiodine resistant metastatic thyroid cancer. Selumetenib 75mg PO BID was given for 4 weeks with the primary outcome being re-induction of RAI avidity. If clinically relevant uptake occurred, the patients were treated with a dose calculated to deliver 2000cGy of ^{131}I to susceptible lesions. Twelve of 20 patients had reinduction of RAI uptake in lesions with 8/12 reaching a threshold considered adequate for treatment. Of those treated, 5/8 had a PR and 3/8 had SD at 6 months of follow up. All patients completed the 4 week course of selumetenib.

Sunitinib(12) – 35 subjects (18 papillary, 5 hürthle cell, 4 follicular, 1 insular, 7 medullary thyroid cancers) were enrolled in a mult-institutional open label study of patients with metastatic radioiodine refractory thyroid cancer. Sunitinib 37.5mg PO QD was initiated and the primary end point was objective response by RECIST criteria. There was one complete remission (CR), 28% of patients had a PR and 46% had stable disease. Median PFS was 12.8 months. No patients went off treatment entirely, but 60% did require at least one 25mg dose reduction secondary to toxicity.

Vandetanib(13) – This was an international, multicenter placebo controlled trial studying the efficacy of vandetanib to increase PFS. 72 patients were randomized to vandetanib 300mg PO QD and 73 matched controls were randomized to placebo. All patients had locally advanced or metastatic radioiodine refractory disease. PFS on vandetanib was 11.1 months as compared to 5.9 months on placebo. No patients discontinued therapy due to adverse toxicity. 38% of patients had dose interruptions and reductions for an average of 18.5 days.

Sorafenib(14-17) – There have been 4 published phase II studies of sorafenib therapy in advanced thyroid cancer. The primary results of all 4 are summarized in Table 2. However, as the only TKI now with an approved indication for advanced DTC, we will go into some depth regarding the US clinical trial data. Sorafenib inhibits human VEGFR 1-3, platelet derived growth factor (PDGF) and RET. The first US trial occurred at the University of Pennsylvania where 30 patients were treated with a starting dose of 400mg BID for a minimum of 16 weeks (14). Twenty-three percent of patients had a partial response lasting more than 18 weeks and 53% of patients had stable disease for up to and beyond 89 weeks. The median progression free survival was 79 weeks. The most common grade 3 (severe but not life-threatening; hospitalization required; limitation of patient's ability to care for him/herself) and grade 4 (Life-threatening; urgent intervention required) toxicities were hypertension (13%), skin rashes (including hand/foot syndrome – a distinct localized cutaneous reaction characterized by erythema, numbness, tingling, and either dysesthesia or paresthesia (18)) (10%) and weight loss (10%). One patient died from acute liver failure that was felt to be treatment related. The second trial occurred at Ohio State University where 56 patients started therapy with 400mg twice daily of sorafenib(15). Patients with metastatic disease from papillary thyroid cancer (PTC) or other DTC histologic subtypes (including four patients with anaplastic thyroid cancer (ATC) were enrolled and had to have measureable disease by Response Evaluation Criteria in Solid Tumors (RECIST) criteria along with radioiodine resistance or were deemed non-RAI candidates by their treating physician(19). Of 41 patients with PTC, 15% had a PR that had a median duration of 7.5 months. Stable disease was observed in 56% of patients for over 6 months. The overall median PFS was 15 months. Progressive disease was noted in 12% of PTC patients despite sorafenib therapy. There were no partial responses seen in patients with non-PTC tumors. Prior treatment with traditional cytotoxic chemotherapy did not yield a significant difference in PFS or overall survival (OS). Dose reduction was required to improve tolerance in 52% of patients. The most common grade 3 adverse events were hand/foot pain (12%), arthralgia (11%) and fatigue (16%). More recently, as reported at the 2013 American Society of Clinical Oncology meeting, the phase III DECISION multi-center trial enrolled 417 patients with progressive DTC refractory to RAI in a randomized placebo controlled fashion (20). The duration of PFS was 10.8 months with sorafenib as compared to 5.8 months with placebo and 12% of patients on sorafenib therapy had a partial response as opposed to <1% of patients in the placebo arm. The study was not powered for overall survival. The occurrence and rates of adverse reactions were similar to previous sorafenib trials. Finally, a recent meta-analysis of trials with sorafenib therapy for advanced thyroid cancer provides broader overview of the benefits and risks of therapy. Overall, 22% of patients treated with Sorafenib achieved a partial response and 52% showed stable disease (with the vast majority of patients having progressive disease prior to enrollment in each trial). Median PFS was 12.4 months when on sorafenib therapy. The most common adverse events associated with sorafenib use were hand-foot syndrome, diarrhea, fatigue, rash, weight loss and hypertension(21).

Table 2

Drug	First Author, Year (Ref.)	N	%PR/%SD	PFS, months
Axitinib	Cohen, 2008 (7)	60	31%/42%	18.1
Gefitinib	Pennell, 2008 (8)	17	0/24%	3.7
Motesanib	Sherman, 2008 (29)	93	14%/67%	9.3
Pazopanib	Bible, 2010 (10)	37	49%/NR	11.7
Selumetenib	Ho, 2013(11)	20	63%/37%	NR
Sorafenib	Gupta-Abramson, 2008(14)	30	23%/53%	21
	Kloos, 2009(15)	41	15%/56%	15
	Hoftijzer, 2009(16)	31	15%/46%	14.5
	Ahmed, 2011(17)	19	16%/74%	16.5
Sunitinib	Carr, 2010 (12)	33	28%/46%	12.8
Vandetanib	Leboulleux, 2012(13)	145 (72 active rx)	8%/57% (on active rx)	11

Published phase II trials of TKI therapy in advanced thyroid cancer. NR= not reported. Adapted from (28) For RECIST criteria--
http://en.wikipedia.org/wiki/Response_Evaluation_Criteria_in_Solid_Tumors

USE IN CLINICAL PRACTICE

At the present time, there are no guidelines detailing how or when TKIs should be used in clinical practice. The most recent American Thyroid Association Thyroid Cancer Guidelines describe TKI use as a future area of research (though they most certainly they will have a more prominent place in the upcoming revised guidelines)(22). Additionally, the most current National Comprehensive Cancer Network guidelines only recommend consideration of TKIs for progressive RAI refractory disease (http://www.nccn.org/professionals/physician_gls/pdf/thyroid.pdf). A recent review of the MD Anderson experience with TKIs and recommendations for use provides rationale guidance in the absence of a consensus multi-center guideline (23). As described in a previous chapter, the selection of an appropriate candidate is likely the most important decision when initiating TKI therapy. Briefly, the current authors would recommend considering patients with at least RAI resistant, unresectable (usually metastatic) disease that is progressive by RECIST criteria for TKI treatment. As opposed to experience in the trials, however, the initiation of TKI therapy for patients with new brain or bone metastases who often were excluded from trials should be considered now that a TKI has been approved for DTC therapy. Practitioners should note, however, that bone metastases in general do not appear to respond as well as, for example, lung metastases (24). Recommendations for pre-initiation assessment include:

1. A detailed history and physical with assessment of the patient's functional status (for example using the Eastern Cooperative Oncology Group performance status (ECOG) (25).
   (http://en.wikipedia.org/wiki/Response_Evaluation_Criteria_in_Solid_Tumors)
   Patients with very poor functional status have generally been denied clinical trial enrollment so their response to therapy is unknown.
2. A comprehensive laboratory analysis assessing metabolic, cardiovascular, hepatic and renal function. Additionally, a baseline electrocardiogram (ECG) is appropriate as TKIs can cause QT prolongation and ECGs should be serially monitored based on the clinical risk (see Figure 1).
3. A detailed discussion with the patient about the expectations of therapy. It is critical to frame the expectations of the patient and physician given the current data ascribed to this class of drugs for the treatment of thyroid cancer. A complete response is extremely unlikely and a partial response can only be expected in 10-20% of patients. The vast majority of patients should expect stabilization of disease for approximately one year (though this may be longer).
4. A detailed explanation of potential side effects is important to help patients avoid unpleasant surprises and allow for earlier symptomatic intervention to attenuate side effects. The most common side effects include(23;26):
   a. Cardiovascular: hypertension, QT prolongation and CHF. All of these should be assessed and optimized prior to starting TKI therapy. Antihypertensive therapy should be individualized for efficacy, tolerance and

cost. ECG should be monitored and significant QT interval prolongation should lead to drug dose reduction or cessation. Electrolytes should be monitored and stabilized as compounding factors and other drugs associated with QT prolongation should be stopped prior to therapy if possible. CHF is rare but patients should be monitored for signs and symptoms at each visit. Baseline cardiac echocardiogram is not unreasonable to have as a comparator for a later study if CHF symptoms present during therapy.

b. Dermatologic manifestations: After diarrhea and fatigue, hand-foot syndrome and other rashes are the most common adverse reactions to TKIs. These usually present early on in therapy and can be treated with creams, emollients, dose reduction or interruption of therapy.

c. Hematologic manifestations: Given the targeting of VEGFR, there is potential bleeding risk with TKIs. These have included issues with thrombocytopenia; poor wound healing and severe bleeding in radiation related fistulas(27).

d. Hepatic manifestations: Side effects have ranged from transient mild transaminitis to fulminant liver failure; though fortunately this has been very rare. Intervention for rising transaminases to 2-3x ULN is generally therapy interruption or cessation.

e. Renal manifestations: Proteinuria has been described with TKI therapy, thus baseline and periodic on treatment urinalyses are appropriate to monitor for this side effect. If significant proteinuria develops, drug cessation is likely necessary.

It is important for prescribing physicians to understand that most TKI trials start with a maximum tolerated dose and a significant subset of patients require dose reductions during the trials. The trial data reported includes those with dose reductions. The authors' experience has been that many patients will require a dose reduction to alleviate side effects, yet tumor responses are consistent with expected and reported outcomes. A common practice in our center is to hold TKI therapy after unacceptable side effects for at least one week or until the side effect resolves, and then reinitiate the medication at 50-75% of the dose depending on the patient and clinician comfort. Should intolerable side effects recur, a second medication hold with re-initiation of medication at 25% of the starting dose is reasonable as long as there is not progressive disease. If there is still intolerance at these dose levels, it is likely time to move on to another therapy. Patients should be reassured that dose reduction will not necessarily translate into a decrease in efficacy, but close observation is critical at lower therapeutic doses.

5. An exploration of costs/payments for these drugs is important as they usually cost thousands of dollars/month. The insurance coverage for sorafenib is likely still being worked out with individual insurers given its recent approval. One clear advantage to clinical trials is the provision of therapy at no cost to the patient.

Finally, most manufacturers have patient assistance programs that should be investigated prior to starting TKI treatment.

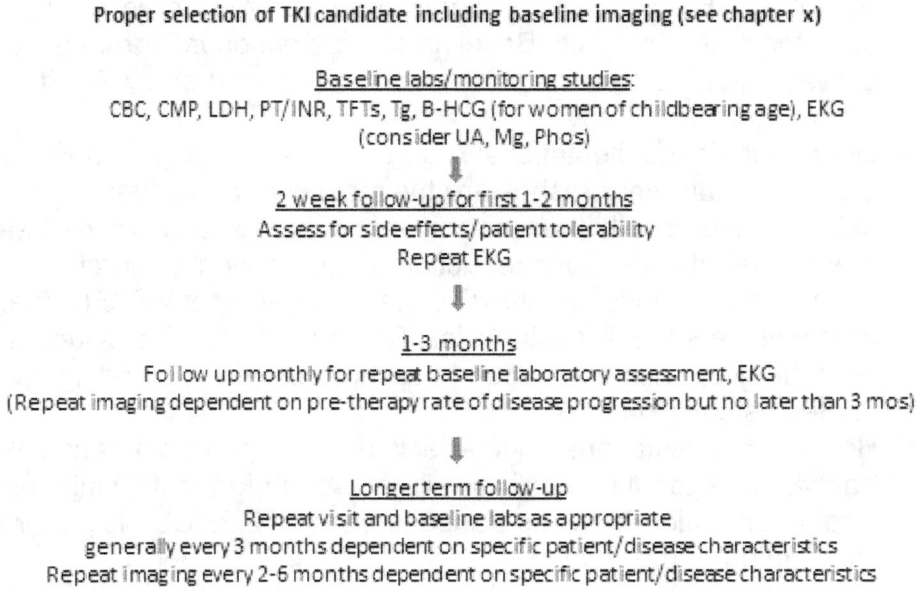

Proper selection of TKI candidate including baseline imaging (see chapter x)

Baseline labs/monitoring studies:
CBC, CMP, LDH, PT/INR, TFTs, Tg, B-HCG (for women of childbearing age), EKG
(consider UA, Mg, Phos)

⬇

2 week follow-up for first 1-2 months
Assess for side effects/patient tolerability
Repeat EKG

⬇

1-3 months
Follow up monthly for repeat baseline laboratory assessment, EKG
(Repeat imaging dependent on pre-therapy rate of disease progression but no later than 3 mos)

⬇

Longer term follow-up
Repeat visit and baseline labs as appropriate
generally every 3 months dependent on specific patient/disease characteristics
Repeat imaging every 2-6 months dependent on specific patient/disease characteristics

Fig 1
Adapted from
(23)

Fig.1

Given that sorafenib is the only approved TKI for metastatic differentiated thyroid cancer at this time, the authors suggest that this should be first line TKI therapy for appropriate candidates. If patients have previously failed sorafenib therapy with progressive disease or intolerance, evaluation of eligible clinical trials is likely the next best option. Finally, off label use of other TKIs with other indications is likely the next most reasonable approach. The TKIs that have been through phase II trials for advanced DTC and are FDA approved for other indications (primarily MTC and advanced renal cell carcinoma) are likely the next best choices. These include vandetanib, sunitinib, pazopanib, axitinib, and gefitinib. Unfortunately, there is no clear correlation between oncoprotein expression (i.e. BRAF) or other molecular marker that can allow for a rationale prediction of one TKI providing more benefit over another based on clinical trial data. Additionally, there has been no trial of combination therapy of TKIs robust enough to lead to a recommendation of combination therapy. Increased toxicity is certainly a significant concern with multi-drug TKI treatment. The choice of TKI therapy after sorafenib may come down to availability, patient preference and comfort level of the treating physician based on their experience with a particular drug.

A very reasonable recommendation for monitoring has been outlined by Carhill et al(23). We believe that after initiation of TKI therapy, clinical and laboratory assessment should be performed at least monthly for the first 3 months along with imaging at 1-3 month intervals dependent on the rate of progression of disease prior to TKI initiation. Seeing a patient back every 2 weeks for the first month or two is reasonable to address concerns over side effects, tolerability and advising on management of side effects. Follow up evaluations should occur at least every 3 months if not more frequently based on the clinical response and tolerability of therapy thereafter. The specific drug package insert should always be checked for monitoring recommendations as post-marketing surveillance may alter such recommendations and drug specific recommendations may be made that do not apply broadly to all available TKIs. Though the typical duration of response will be approximately one year, patients should stay on prescribed therapy in the absence of progressive disease for as long as possible. It is important to note, progression at any point on one TKI does not necessarily predict failure of another TKI. This is likely attributable to the numerous targets and pathways these medications inhibit with different TKIs having overlapping and unique targets. When a patient has failed multiple TKI therapies (or not tolerated them), and there is rapid progression of disease, consideration of chemotherapy or phase I clinical trials is appropriate. An overall diagram of initiating and monitoring therapy is proposed in figure 1.

Finally, as described in the phase II trial data above, novel indications for TKI therapy in thyroid cancer are currently being investigated. The most exciting recent development has been the discovery that the TKI selumetenib appears to induce re-differentiation of RAI resistant thyroid cancers to be able to concentrate sufficient RAI for therapeutic benefit (11). There are now two multicenter studies studying the use of selumetenib in thyroid cancer. One is functionally an expansion of the aforementioned trial, while the other is a unique approach using selumetenib as a neo-adjuvant agent prior to initial 131I therapy in patients with aggressive localized disease.

In summary, the dissection of molecular pathways and events leading to the propagation of cancers of many types, including thyroid cancer, has led to a dramatic expansion of oral, targeted, generally well tolerated therapies for advanced malignancies. As opposed to cytotoxic chemotherapies that have historically had an unacceptable side effects and minimal therapeutic benefit in advanced DTC, TKIs have opened the door for at least bridge therapy for patients with progressive metastatic thyroid cancer while new therapeutic discoveries continue.

Reference List

1. O'Neill CJ, Oucharek J, Learoyd D, Sidhu SB. Standard and emerging therapies for metastatic differentiated thyroid cancer. Oncologist 2010; 15(2):146-156.

2. Dupuy DE, Monchik JM, Decrea C, Pisharodi L. Radiofrequency ablation of regional recurrence from well-differentiated thyroid malignancy. Surgery 2001; 130(6):971-977.

3. Lewis BD, Hay ID, Charboneau JW, McIver B, Reading CC, Goellner JR. Percutaneous ethanol injection for treatment of cervical lymph node metastases in patients with papillary thyroid carcinoma. AJR Am J Roentgenol 2002; 178(3):699-704.

4. Magarey MJ, Freeman JL. Recurrent well-differentiated thyroid carcinoma. Oral Oncol 2013; 49(7):689-694.

5. Haugen BR, Sherman SI. Evolving approaches to patients with advanced differentiated thyroid cancer. Endocr Rev 2013; 34(3):439-455.

6. Brose M. Sorafenib in locally advanced or metastatic patients with radioactive iodine-refractory differentiated thyroid cancer: The phase III DECISION trial. Nutting C, Jarzab B, Elisei R et al., editors. Journal of Clinical Oncology 31[18], 4. 6-20-0013.
Ref Type: Abstract

7. Cohen EE, Rosen LS, Vokes EE et al. Axitinib is an active treatment for all histologic subtypes of advanced thyroid cancer: results from a phase II study. J Clin Oncol 2008; 26(29):4708-4713.

8. Pennell NA, Daniels GH, Haddad RI et al. A phase II study of gefitinib in patients with advanced thyroid cancer. Thyroid 2008; 18(3):317-323.

9. Sherman SI, Wirth LJ, Droz JP et al. Motesanib diphosphate in progressive differentiated thyroid cancer. N Engl J Med 2008; 359(1):31-42.

10. Bible KC, Suman VJ, Molina JR et al. Efficacy of pazopanib in progressive, radioiodine-refractory, metastatic differentiated thyroid cancers: results of a phase 2 consortium study. Lancet Oncol 2010; 11(10):962-972.

11. Ho AL, Grewal RK, Leboeuf R et al. Selumetinib-enhanced radioiodine uptake in advanced thyroid cancer. N Engl J Med 2013; 368(7):623-632.

12. Carr LL, Mankoff DA, Goulart BH et al. Phase II study of daily sunitinib in FDG-PET-positive, iodine-refractory differentiated thyroid cancer and metastatic medullary

carcinoma of the thyroid with functional imaging correlation. Clin Cancer Res 2010; 16(21):5260-5268.

13. Leboulleux S, Bastholt L, Krause T et al. Vandetanib in locally advanced or metastatic differentiated thyroid cancer: a randomised, double-blind, phase 2 trial. Lancet Oncol 2012; 13(9):897-905.

14. Gupta-Abramson V, Troxel AB, Nellore A et al. Phase II trial of sorafenib in advanced thyroid cancer. J Clin Oncol 2008; 26(29):4714-4719.

15. Kloos RT, Ringel MD, Knopp MV et al. Phase II trial of sorafenib in metastatic thyroid cancer. J Clin Oncol 2009; 27(10):1675-1684.

16. Hoftijzer H, Heemstra KA, Morreau H et al. Beneficial effects of sorafenib on tumor progression, but not on radioiodine uptake, in patients with differentiated thyroid carcinoma. Eur J Endocrinol 2009; 161(6):923-931.

17. Ahmed M, Barbachano Y, Riddell A et al. Analysis of the efficacy and toxicity of sorafenib in thyroid cancer: a phase II study in a UK based population. Eur J Endocrinol 2011; 165(2):315-322.

18. Chu D, Lacouture ME, Fillos T, Wu S. Risk of hand-foot skin reaction with sorafenib: a systematic review and meta-analysis. Acta Oncol 2008; 47(2):176-186.

19. Ganten MK, Ganten TM, Schlemmer HP. Radiological Monitoring of the Treatment of Solid Tumors in Practice. Rofo 2014.

20. Brose MS, Nutting CM, Sherman SI et al. Rationale and design of decision: a double-blind, randomized, placebo-controlled phase III trial evaluating the efficacy and safety of sorafenib in patients with locally advanced or metastatic radioactive iodine (RAI)-refractory, differentiated thyroid cancer. BMC Cancer 2011; 11:349.

21. Shen CT, Qiu Z, Luo QY. Sorafenib in radioiodine-refractory differentiated thyroid cancer: a meta-analysis. Endocr Relat Cancer 2013.

22. Cooper DS, Doherty GM, Haugen BR et al. Revised American Thyroid Association management guidelines for patients with thyroid nodules and differentiated thyroid cancer. Thyroid 2009; 19(11):1167-1214.

23. Carhill AA, Cabanillas ME, Jimenez C et al. The noninvestigational use of tyrosine kinase inhibitors in thyroid cancer: establishing a standard for patient safety and monitoring. J Clin Endocrinol Metab 2013; 98(1):31-42.

24. Cabanillas ME, Waguespack SG, Bronstein Y et al. Treatment with tyrosine kinase inhibitors for patients with differentiated thyroid cancer: the M. D. Anderson experience. J Clin Endocrinol Metab 2010; 95(6):2588-2595.

25. Oken MM, Creech RH, Tormey DC et al. Toxicity and response criteria of the Eastern Cooperative Oncology Group. Am J Clin Oncol 1982; 5(6):649-655.

26. Cabanillas ME, Hu MI, Durand JB, Busaidy NL. Challenges associated with tyrosine kinase inhibitor therapy for metastatic thyroid cancer. J Thyroid Res 2011; 2011:985780.

27. Kirkali Z. Adverse events from targeted therapies in advanced renal cell carcinoma: the impact on long-term use. BJU Int 2011; 107(11):1722-1732.

28. Haraldsdottir S, Shah MH. An update on clinical trials of targeted therapies in thyroid cancer. Curr Opin Oncol 2014; 26(1):36-44.

29. Sherman SI, Wirth LJ, Droz JP et al. Motesanib diphosphate in progressive differentiated thyroid cancer. N Engl J Med 2008; 359(1):31-42.

S5-FUTURE DIRECTIONS IN THERAPY OF ADVANCED THYROID CANCER.

James A. Fagin[1,2] and Alan Ho [2]
Human Oncology and Pathogenesis Program[1] and Department of Medicine[2], Memorial Sloan-Kettering Cancer Center, New York, NY.

THE EXPERIENCE WITH MULTIKINASE INHIBITORS:

The primary emphasis in experimental therapeutics of advanced thyroid cancer over the past decade has been on testing the effectiveness of ATP-competitive multikinase small molecule inhibitors. These are thought to act mostly by inhibiting receptor tyrosine kinases such as VEGFR and PDGFR, which play an important role in tumor neovascularization. Although sorafenib is the only member of this class that is FDA-approved for treatment of follicular cell-derived thyroid cancer, several others, such as pazopanib, lenvatinib, motesanib and vandetanib, have also shown clinical benefit, manifesting as RECIST-confirmed partial responses and extension of progression-free survival (1). It is unclear whether these compounds act entirely through their effects on the tumor microenvironment, or whether they also exert direct growth inhibitory effects on the cancer cells, and if so, through which mechanisms.

Sorafenib inhibits RAF kinase activity *in vitro*, but is unlikely to achieve therapeutically significant inhibitory effects on oncogenic BRAF in patients because of the narrow therapeutic window of the compound. In this respect, one key lesson from the experience of treating patients with metastatic BRAF-mutant melanomas is that clinical efficacy requires inhibiting BRAF kinase activity in a profound and sustained manner, which can be achieved with compounds that are highly selective, such as vemurafenib (2) or dabrafenib. By contrast sorafenib was ineffective as a monotherapy in patients with BRAF-mutant melanoma (3).

Other drugs, such as vandetanib and lenvatinib, have been proposed to have cancer cell intrinsic inhibitory effects by targeting EGFR. There is no evidence that EGFR is a primary driver of the disease, as *EGFR* mutations and gene amplification are rarely, if ever, present (4). Moreover, a small trial of gefitinib showed very modest effects in patients with metastatic thyroid cancer (5).

Despite evidence for clinical benefit, we still don't know whether multikinase inhibitors prolong overall survival of patients with advanced thyroid cancer. One corollary of the experience with this class of compounds in thyroid cancer is that they do not truly represent examples of personalized therapies, since the genetic characteristics of the tumor do not predict clinical responses. The specific proteins or pathways targeted by these drugs that are critical for clinical activity have not been clearly established. Although these agents inhibit overlapping molecular targets, different inhibitors within this class can still induce responses in the salvage setting following sorafenib failure (6), possibly due to the existence of non-redundant targets and/or differences in the therapeutic window for each drug. Promising results are being reported with combinations involving multikinase inhibitors and other targeted agents (e.g., mTOR inhibitors), without definitive insights into how these agents interact to augment clinical responses. Without a better understanding of their mechanism of action, it will continue to be difficult to envision how to rationally design new treatment paradigms with these compounds.

THE ROLE OF CYTOTOXIC CHEMOTHERAPY AGENTS:

The emerging role of molecular targeted therapies for treating thyroid cancer raises the question regarding the relevance of cytotoxic chemotherapy agents for managing this disease. Until the recent FDA-approval of sorafenib, doxorubicin was the only systemic agent approved for the treatment of thyroid cancer (7). The concern regarding cytotoxic drugs such as doxorubicin, paclitaxel, and cisplatin is that the limited published studies report only modest response rates and short durations of therapeutic benefit. Nonetheless, these drugs are still acceptable options for patients who cannot tolerate treatment with multikinase inhibitors or who have relative contraindications to the use of anti-angiogenic therapies, such as the existence of active bleeding (e.g., hemoptysis). Anaplastic thyroid cancer is an aggressive, rapidly progressive disease for which multikinase inhibitors have no significant clinical efficacy (8). Currently, cytotoxic agents remain the only viable systemic option (9). Given the genetic complexity of anaplastic thyroid cancer and the clinical need to induce tumor responses rapidly, this is the thyroid cancer subtype in which cytotoxic chemotherapy will likely continue to be a relevant part of future investigational approaches, primarily in combination with molecular targeted therapies. For instance, recent gene expression profiling of anaplastic thyroid cancers in mouse models revealed the presence of a deregulated "mitotic signature" in addition to the canonical "driver" mutations that result in constitutive MAPK pathway activation (e.g., mutant *BRAF*, *RAS*, and others) (10). This biology suggests that combinations of a cytotoxic that can elicit mitotic arrest (e.g., paclitaxel) with a MAPK pathway targeted therapy may be worth testing for anaplastic thyroid cancer.

Cytotoxic chemotherapy may also be used as a radiosensitizer for external beam radiation therapy applied to locally advanced or recurrent thyroid cancer. Retrospective studies show that radiation combined with doxorubicin can elicit effective locoregional control for locally-advanced, follicular-cell derived thyroid carcinomas (11) and to a lesser extent anaplastic thyroid cancer (12). An area of active investigation is how molecular targeted agents alone or in combination with cytotoxic chemotherapy may elicit more effective and durable locoregional control when administered concurrently with radiation therapy.

TARGETING THE GENETIC DRIVERS OF THYROID CANCER:

The Cancer Genome Atlas (TCGA) program recently completed a comprehensive genomic analysis of approximately 500 papillary thyroid cancers (PTC), which largely confirms prior studies regarding the frequency of the key driver mutations in the disease: *BRAF* 57%, *RAS* 12% and fusion oncogenes (*RET/PTC*, *NTRK1*, *BRAF*, others) 9%, which are all mutually exclusive. These mutations are all effectors in the MAPK signaling pathway, the activation of which was confirmed through RNA sequencing, which showed robust induction of components of the MAPK transcriptional output (13), as well as by analysis of specific members of the phosphoproteome. *BRAF* mutations are found in classical and tall cell variant PTCs, whereas *RAS* mutations are highly prevalent in follicular variant PTCs, consistent with prior reports (14;15). The molecular taxonomy is different in advanced disease. Thus, although poorly differentiated (PDTC) and anaplastic thyroid cancers (ATC) also frequently harbor *BRAF* mutations, they are comparatively enriched for *RAS* mutations: 23-44% in PDTC (16;17) and 22% in ATC (18).

There is ample preclinical evidence that thyroid cancers retain dependency for viability on the constitutive activity of the oncogenic driver responsible for tumor development. This has been established in mouse models of *Braf*-mutant papillary thyroid cancers (19;20), and is consistent with a paradigm that is now well accepted in oncology. Therapeutic targeting of oncoproteins such as BCR-ABL in chronic myelogenous leukemia (21;22), KIT in gastrointestinal stromal tumors (23), mutant EGFR in non-small cell lung cancer (24), and BRAF in metastatic melanomas (25;26) induces cancer cell apoptosis and major clinical responses. These concepts and strategies are only just beginning to be applied in clinical trials for patients with advanced thyroid cancers.

ENHANCING EFFECTIVENESS OF RADIOIODINE THERAPY BY INHIBITION OF MAPK SIGNALING:

The natural history of metastatic thyroid cancer is often marked by a prolonged period of asymptomatic insidious disease progression. The only treatment option available to these patients in the past was radioiodine, which was often given repeatedly despite lack of evidence for benefit, as many patients with metastatic thyroid cancer have tumors that do not incorporate iodine efficiently. This is associated with worse prognosis: i.e. the 10-year survival of patients with metastatic thyroid cancer that retains RAI avidity is ~60%, whereas it is only 10% if the metastases are refractory to RAI therapy (27). Oncogenic activation of MAPK signaling in thyroid cells leads to loss of expression of genes required for thyroid hormone biosynthesis, including the sodium iodide transporter (NIS) and thyroid peroxidase (TPO) (28;29). The activating BRAF^{V600E} mutation is the most frequent genetic alteration in PTC (30-32) and confers a comparatively worse prognosis (30;33-36). Tumors with *BRAF* mutation have lower expression of NIS (37), which likely explains the clinical observation that *BRAF* mutant PTCs are often particularly resistant to RAI therapy.

Mouse models of thyroid cancer driven by oncogenic BRAF develop tumors that recapitulate the observations in patients, in that they lose the ability to concentrate radioiodine. Moreover, when the activation of BRAF is switched off genetically, or its downstream signaling is targeted with small molecule kinase inhibitors of RAF or MEK, the tumors regain the ability to trap radioiodine (19). The experiments performed in mice provided the rationale for a pilot clinical trial in which patients with RAI-refractory metastatic thyroid cancer were treated with the MEK inhibitor selumetinib (AZD6244; AstraZeneca), in an attempt to restore RAI responsiveness. Briefly, patients known to have RAI-refractory distant metastatic disease underwent ^{124}I PET scans after stimulation with recombinant TSH before and again after receiving a 4-week course of selumetinib. ^{124}I is a positron-emitting isotope, which allows precise quantification of uptake in the metastatic lesions. Altogether, 12 of the 20 evaluable patients had marked increased uptake on the ^{124}I-PET scans after treatment with the drug. Eight of these patients (8/20; 40%) had lesional uptakes that by dosimetry predicted that an effective dose of $\geq$2,000 cGy of ^{131}I could be delivered, and they were therefore treated with a therapeutic dose of ^{131}I. In these patients, the metastatic tumors decreased in size and the thyroglobulin levels, which serve as an effective biomarker for the disease, decreased dramatically. The responses were particularly striking in patients whose tumors harbored *RAS* mutations, whereas patients with *BRAF*-mutant disease had a more attenuated response (38). As discussed below, elucidation of the mechanisms accounting for the relative refractoriness of *BRAF*-mutant thyroid cancers to MEK and RAF kinase inhibitors provide promising strategies to improve on these outcomes.

OVERCOMING ADAPTIVE RESISTANCE TO RAF AND MEK INHIBITORS IN BRAF-MUTANT THYROID CANCERS:

By contrast to the high response rate seen in patients with metastatic melanomas (25;26), the RAF kinase inhibitor vemurafenib has limited efficacy as a single agent in patients with *BRAF*-mutant colorectal cancers (39). A clinical trial evaluating vemurafenib in *BRAF*-mutant thyroid cancer patients was recently completed, and presented in a late-breaking abstract by Marcia Brose at the European Cancer Organization's (ECCO) 2013 European Cancer Congress. A 35% response rate was seen in patients not previously treated with multikinase inhibitors. Although encouraging, this rate of response is of a lesser magnitude than what has been reported for patients with metastatic melanoma. Hence, although cancers of these three lineages (i.e. colon, melanoma and thyroid) harbor the same genetic driver, they differ in their response to a selective and highly effective inhibitor of mutant BRAF kinase.

Activation of MAPK signaling in non-transformed cells occurs in response to growth factors, cytokines and stress signals. BRAF-transformed cells hyperactivate MAPK independently of upstream inputs, to which cells become unresponsive through engagement of ERK-dependent negative feedback loops (40). Accordingly, RAS-GTP levels are depleted in *BRAF*-mutant tumor cells regardless of their cell type, and the activation state of receptor tyrosine kinases (RTKs) is low. When exposed to RAF or MEK inhibitors the signaling network of BRAF-mutant melanoma and thyroid cancer cells adapts by relaxing the repression of upstream signaling inputs, although they do so to a different extent depending in large part on the cell type. By contrast to melanomas, thyroid cells show rapid and robust increases in RAS-GTP shortly after exposure to RAF kinase inhibitors, due in large part to activation of HER3/HER2 signaling. This is caused by induction of HER3 and HER2 transcription, through decreased HER3 and HER2 promoter occupancy by the transcriptional repressors CtBP1 and 2. As BRAF-mutant thyroid cancer also constitutively secrete the HER3 ligand neuregulin-1, they are primed to reactivate signaling, which dampens responses to inhibition of mutant BRAF (41). The HER family kinase inhibitor lapatinib prevents MAPK rebound and sensitizes BRAF-mutant thyroid cancer cells to RAF or MEK inhibitors. This provides a rationale for combining inhibitors of the ERK pathway with inhibitors of feedback-reactivated HER signaling in this disease, and a phase I clinical trial with a combination of dabrafenib and lapatinib is currently in progress to test this hypothesis in patients.

Interestingly, patients with BRAF-mutant colorectal cancer are mostly unresponsive to the RAF inhibitor vemurafenib. The mechanisms of adaptive resistance to RAF kinase inhibitors in colorectal cancers is similar, but distinct, from that of thyroid cancer cells. It has recently been ascribed to activation of epidermal growth factor receptor (EGFR) signaling (42;43), due to feedback-induced relaxation of the activity of CDC25C, a putative EGFR phosphatase (42). Hence, although RTK induction may be ubiquitous in response to MAPK pathway inhibition, the determinants of adaptive resistance vary between cancer types. This is due to preferential upregulation of specific RTKs in different cancer cell lineages, and is also likely to be critically dependent on the abundance of their respective ligands in the cancer microenvironment, either through autocrine production or from other sources.

The reactivation of MAPK through RTKs or through derepression of wild-type RAS activity in response to RAF kinase inhibitors converges through MEK. Hence, combined therapy with RAF and MEK kinase inhibitors is a rational approach to overcome adaptive resistance. A combination of dabrafenib and trametinib was recently granted accelerated approval by the FDA for patients with metastatic BRAF^{V00E} melanoma (44), and will soon be tested in patients with BRAF-mutant thyroid cancer.

ACQUIRED RESISTANCE TO RAF OR MEK INHIBITORS:

Patients whose cancers respond initially to inhibitors of the oncogenic driver of the disease (e.g. BRAF^{V600E} melanoma to vemurafenib, EGFR-mutant non-small cell lung cancer to gefitinib) often find that these responses are not durable because of emergence of acquired resistance. About 50% of patients with *EGFR*-mutant lung adenocarcinomas that develop resistance to gefitinib or erlotinib acquire a second site mutation in *EGFR* that substitutes methionine for threonine at position 790 (T790M), the so-called "gatekeeper residue", and which renders the receptor unresponsive to first line EGFR inhibitors. This paradigm, which recapitulates mechanisms of resistance to other selective kinase inhibitors (e.g. to imatinib in BCR-ABL mutant CML and KIT mutant GIST), provides further proof for the dependence of the tumor clone on the activity of the oncogenic driver for viability. In the case of BRAF-mutant cancers, the largest experience so far is in patients with metastatic melanomas treated with vemurafenib. Acquired resistance occurs through selection of resistant clones that harbor activating mutations of *RAS* or MEK1, or that express a splice variant of BRAF, p61BRAF(V600E), which lacks exons 4–8, a region that encompasses the RAS-binding domain, and which shows enhanced dimerization that confers resistance to the inhibitor (45). There is no information so far on acquired resistance in the context of *BRAF*-mutant thyroid cancers. In those tumors that show a primary response to RAF inhibitors, resistance is likely to occur sooner or later. If and when they do, it will be important to define the mechanisms of resistance in biopsy material of lesions that progress while on therapy, since these will guide the design of combination therapies that may induce more sustained clinical responses.

A commonly stated concern is whether tumors that have a severely disrupted genome will still respond to selective therapies directed against a single oncoprotein. Patients with BRAF-mutant metastatic melanoma harbor lesions with a very high overall burden of mutations (46), and yet, as mentioned, have remarkable responses to RAF kinase inhibitors. A recent case report documented striking regression of the disease following treatment of a patient with BRAF-mutant anaplastic thyroid cancer with lung metastases with vemurafenib (47), suggesting that even this extraordinarily virulent malignancy may remain dependent for survival on the primary oncogenic driver.

TARGETING OTHER ONCOGENIC DRIVERS OF THYROID CANCER:

Most advanced cases of thyroid cancer harbor mutations of either BRAF or RAS. However, a significant fraction of metastatic thyroid cancers are driven by other mutant oncoproteins. Many of these, such as rearrangements of RET, ALK, NRTK1 or 3 are potentially drug-treatable. Despite their relative rarity, new approaches to trial design should now enable investigation of whether kinase inhibitors with activity against these mutant fusion oncoproteins provide clinical benefit. Other than for phase I studies, the conventional design of experimental therapeutic trials in oncology have been almost entirely disease-focused. Based on the strong evidence supporting the value of targeted therapies, trials can now be designed against mutant oncoproteins across disease types. This approach, which has been termed "basket trial", enrolls patients with cancers harboring mutations of a specific oncoprotein on a treatment protocol with a drug that targets its activity, with each "basket" corresponding to a particular disease type (48). For instance, for a hypothetical basket trial of a drug targeting FGFR fusions, one basket could be for patients with bladder cancer, another for lung, another for thyroid, etc. A relatively small number of patients can be enrolled in each basket, allowing for simultaneous investigation of the role of the driver in different lineages. If activity is seen in one or more particular entity, that cohort can be expanded to allow for more meaningful conclusions. It is now conceivable that regulatory agencies may consider accelerated approval for drugs tested in this manner if the rationale is compelling, the results are clear and there is an unmet need.

CANCER IMMUNOTHERAPIES:

Rationally designed strategies targeting oncogenes and/or their signaling cascades are clinically effective, but the almost inevitable development of either adaptive and/or acquired resistance has precluded durable tumor responses in most patients. A new generation of immunotherapies has emerged that target negative regulatory receptors on T cells. Ipilimumab, the prototypic monoclonal antibody of this class, blocks the cytotoxic T cell receptor-4 (CTLA-4) on activated T cells (49). CTLA-4 is latently expressed on activated T cells during acute inflammation. Engagement of CTLA-4 by its ligand B7, expressed primarily on antigen presenting cells, suppresses T cell proliferation and helps restore tissue homeostasis. The clinical efficacy of targeting CTLA-4 in patients with metastatic melanoma was established in a milestone phase III clinical trial in which ipilimumab improved the overall survival of patients from 6.4 months to 10 months. Several patients exhibited complete responses that lasted for years. The results of this study led to the FDA approval of ipilimumab for patients with metastatic melanoma in 2011. A second emerging immunoregulatory target is the programmed cell death-1 (PD-1) receptor, which is expressed on hematopoietic cells, including T cells (50). The ligands for the receptor, PD-L1 and PD-L2, are expressed by antigen presenting cells, inflamed tissues, as well as by tumor cells, including thyroid cancers (51). Binding of PD-1 by PD-L1 or PD-L2 negatively regulates activated cytotoxic T cell functions and provides an additional mechanism by which tumors escape anti-tumor immunity. PD-1 blocking antibodies are showing remarkably durable responses in a number of tumor types, including lung, prostate, melanoma and others. The possible cooperation between these dual negative T cell checkpoint regulators on the adaptive immune response is also currently being explored in clinical trials with combined anti-CTLA-4 and anti-PD-1 blockade in patients with metastatic melanoma. These approaches have not yet been tested in thyroid cancer, but there is reason to believe that they may hold significant potential, since anti-thyroid autoimmune responses were noted in patients with metastatic melanoma treated with ipilimumab (52). Based on these and other recent breakthroughs in cancer immunotherapy (53) clinical trials will need to re-evaluate approaches that are based solely on the genetic characteristics of the tumors, and consider the place that each strategy, alone or in combination, may have in the treatment of different tumor types, including thyroid cancer.

Acknowledgements: Supported by NIH grants CA50706 and CA72597. The authors gratefully acknowledge generous gifts from the Society of Memorial Sloan Kettering, the Byrne, J Randolph Hearst and the Lefkovsky Family Foundations.

Reference List

1. Sherman,S.I. 2011. Targeted therapies for thyroid tumors. *Mod. Pathol.* 24 Suppl 2:S44-52.:S44-S52.

2. Bollag,G., Hirth,P., Tsai,J., Zhang,J., Ibrahim,P.N., Cho,H., Spevak,W., Zhang,C., Zhang,Y., Habets,G. et al 2010. Clinical efficacy of a RAF inhibitor needs broad target blockade in BRAF-mutant melanoma. *Nature.* 467:596-599.

3. Eisen,T., Ahmad,T., Flaherty,K.T., Gore,M., Kaye,S., Marais,R., Gibbens,I., Hackett,S., James,M., Schuchter,L.M. et al 2006. Sorafenib in advanced melanoma: a Phase II randomised discontinuation trial analysis. *Br. J Cancer.* 95:581-586.

4. Ricarte-Filho,J.C., Matsuse,M., Lau,C., Ryder,M., Nishihara,E., Ghossein,R.A., Ladanyi,M., Yamashita,S., Mitsutake,N., and Fagin,J.A. 2011. Absence of common activating mutations of the epidermal growth factor receptor gene in thyroid cancers from American and Japanese patients. *Int. J. Cancer.*10.

5. Pennell,N.A., Daniels,G.H., Haddad,R.I., Ross,D.S., Evans,T., Wirth,L.J., Fidias,P.H., Temel,J.S., Gurubhagavatula,S., Heist,R.S. et al 2008. A phase II study of gefitinib in patients with advanced thyroid cancer. *THYROID.* 18:317-323.

6. Dadu,R., Devine,C., Hernandez,M., Waguespack,S.G., Busaidy,N.L., Hu,M.I., Jimenez,C., Habra,M.A., Sellin,R.V., Ying,A.K. et al 2014. Role of salvage targeted therapy in differentiated thyroid cancer patients who failed first-line sorafenib. *J. Clin. Endocrinol. Metab.*jc20133588.

7. Shimaoka,K., Schoenfeld,D.A., DeWys,W.D., Creech,R.H., and DeConti,R. 1985. A randomized trial of doxorubicin versus doxorubicin plus cisplatin in patients with advanced thyroid carcinoma. *Cancer.* 56:2155-2160.

8. Bible,K.C., Suman,V.J., Menefee,M.E., Smallridge,R.C., Molina,J.R., Maples,W.J., Karlin,N.J., Traynor,A.M., Kumar,P., Goh,B.C. et al 2012. A multiinstitutional phase 2 trial of pazopanib monotherapy in advanced anaplastic thyroid cancer. *J. Clin. Endocrinol. Metab.* 97:3179-3184.

9. Ain,K.B., Egorin,M.J., and DeSimone,P.A. 2000. Treatment of anaplastic thyroid carcinoma with paclitaxel: phase 2 trial using ninety-six-hour infusion. Collaborative Anaplastic Thyroid Cancer Health Intervention Trials (CATCHIT) Group. *THYROID.* 10:587-594.

10. Russo,M.A., Kang,K.S., and Di Cristofano,A. 2013. The PLK1 inhibitor GSK461364A is effective in poorly differentiated and anaplastic thyroid carcinoma cells, independent of the nature of their driver mutations. *THYROID.* 23:1284-1293.

11. Kim,J.H., and Leeper,R.D. 1987. Treatment of locally advanced thyroid carcinoma with combination doxorubicin and radiation therapy. *Cancer.* 60:2372-2375.

12. Sherman,E.J., Lim,S.H., Ho,A.L., Ghossein,R.A., Fury,M.G., Shaha,A.R., Rivera,M., Lin,O., Wolden,S., Lee,N.Y. et al 2011. Concurrent doxorubicin and radiotherapy for anaplastic thyroid cancer: a critical re-evaluation including uniform pathologic review. *Radiother. Oncol.* 101:425-430.

13. Pratilas,C.A., Taylor,B.S., Ye,Q., Viale,A., Sander,C., Solit,D.B., and Rosen,N. 2009. (V600E)BRAF is associated with disabled feedback inhibition of RAF-MEK signaling and elevated transcriptional output of the pathway. *Proc. Natl. Acad. Sci. U. S. A.* 106:4519-4524.

14. Zhu,Z., Gandhi,M., Nikiforova,M.N., Fischer,A.H., and Nikiforov,Y.E. 2003. Molecular profile and clinical-pathologic features of the follicular variant of papillary thyroid carcinoma. An unusually high prevalence of ras mutations. *Am. J. Clin. Pathol.* 120:71-77.

15. Rivera,M., Ricarte-Filho,J., Knauf,J., Shaha,A., Tuttle,M., Fagin,J.A., and Ghossein,R.A. 2010. Molecular genotyping of papillary thyroid carcinoma follicular variant according to its histological subtypes (encapsulated vs infiltrative) reveals distinct BRAF and RAS mutation patterns. *Mod. Pathol.* 23:1191-1200.

16. Volante,M., Rapa,I., Gandhi,M., Bussolati,G., Giachino,D., Papotti,M., and Nikiforov,Y.E. 2009. RAS mutations are the predominant molecular alteration in poorly differentiated thyroid carcinomas and bear prognostic impact. *J. Clin. Endocrinol. Metab.* 94:4735-4741.

17. Ricarte-Filho,J.C., Ryder,M., Chitale,D.A., Rivera,M., Heguy,A., Ladanyi,M., Janakiraman,M., Solit,D., Knauf,J.A., Tuttle,R.M. et al 2009. Mutational profile of advanced primary and metastatic radioactive iodine-refractory thyroid cancers reveals distinct pathogenetic roles for BRAF, PIK3CA, and AKT1. *Cancer Res.* 69:4885-4893.

18. Smallridge,R.C., Marlow,L.A., and Copland,J.A. 2009. Anaplastic thyroid cancer: molecular pathogenesis and emerging therapies. *Endocr. Relat Cancer.* 16:17-44.

19. Chakravarty,D., Santos,E., Ryder,M., Knauf,J.A., Liao,X.H., West,B.L., Bollag,G., Kolesnick,R., Thin,T.H., Rosen,N. et al 2011. Small-molecule MAPK inhibitors restore radioiodine incorporation in mouse thyroid cancers with conditional BRAF activation. *J. Clin. Invest.* 121:4700-4711.

20. Charles,R.P., Iezza,G., Amendola,E., Dankort,D., and McMahon,M. 2011. Mutationally activated BRAF(V600E) elicits papillary thyroid cancer in the adult mouse. *Cancer Res.* 71:3863-3871.

21. Druker,B.J., Talpaz,M., Resta,D.J., Peng,B., Buchdunger,E., Ford,J.M., Lydon,N.B., Kantarjian,H., Capdeville,R., Ohno-Jones,S. et al 2001. Efficacy and safety of a specific inhibitor of the BCR-ABL tyrosine kinase in chronic myeloid leukemia. *N. Engl. J. Med.* 344:1031-1037.

22. Sawyers,C.L., Hochhaus,A., Feldman,E., Goldman,J.M., Miller,C.B., Ottmann,O.G., Schiffer,C.A., Talpaz,M., Guilhot,F., Deininger,M.W. et al 2002. Imatinib induces hematologic and cytogenetic responses in patients with chronic myelogenous leukemia in myeloid blast crisis: results of a phase II study. *Blood.* 99:3530-3539.

23. Heinrich,M.C., Corless,C.L., Demetri,G.D., Blanke,C.D., von Mehren,M., Joensuu,H., McGreevey,L.S., Chen,C.J., Van den Abbeele,A.D., Druker,B.J. et al 2003. Kinase mutations and imatinib response in patients with metastatic gastrointestinal stromal tumor. *J. Clin. Oncol.* 21:4342-4349.

24. Lynch,T.J., Bell,D.W., Sordella,R., Gurubhagavatula,S., Okimoto,R.A., Brannigan,B.W., Harris,P.L., Haserlat,S.M., Supko,J.G., Haluska,F.G. et al 2004. Activating mutations in the epidermal growth factor receptor underlying responsiveness of non-small-cell lung cancer to gefitinib. *N. Engl. J. Med.* %20;350:2129-2139.

25. Chapman,P.B., Hauschild,A., Robert,C., Haanen,J.B., Ascierto,P., Larkin,J., Dummer,R., Garbe,C., Testori,A., Maio,M. et al 2011. Improved survival with vemurafenib in melanoma with BRAF V600E mutation. *N. Engl. J. Med.* 364:2507-2516.

26. Flaherty,K.T., Puzanov,I., Kim,K.B., Ribas,A., McArthur,G.A., Sosman,J.A., O'dwyer,P.J., Lee,R.J., Grippo,J.F., Nolop,K. et al 2010. Inhibition of mutated, activated BRAF in metastatic melanoma. *N. Engl. J. Med.* 363:809-819.

27. Durante,C., Haddy,N., Baudin,E., Leboulleux,S., Hartl,D., Travagli,J.P., Caillou,B., Ricard,M., Lumbroso,J.D., De,V.F. et al 2006. Long-term outcome of 444 patients with distant metastases from papillary and follicular thyroid carcinoma: benefits and limits of radioiodine therapy. *J. Clin. Endocrinol. Metab.* 91:2892-2899.

28. Knauf,J.A., Kuroda,H., Basu,S., and Fagin,J.A. 2003. RET/PTC-induced dedifferentiation of thyroid cells is mediated through Y1062 signaling through SHC-RAS-MAP kinase. *Oncogene* 22:4406-4412.

29. Mitsutake,N., Knauf,J.A., Mitsutake,S., Mesa,C., Jr., Zhang,L., and Fagin,J.A. 2005. Conditional BRAFV600E expression induces DNA synthesis, apoptosis, dedifferentiation, and chromosomal instability in thyroid PCCL3 cells. *Cancer Res.* 65:2465-2473.

30. Kimura,E.T., Nikiforova,M.N., Zhu,Z., Knauf,J.A., Nikiforov,Y.E., and Fagin,J.A. 2003. High prevalence of BRAF mutations in thyroid cancer: genetic evidence for constitutive activation of the RET/PTC-RAS-BRAF signaling pathway in papillary thyroid carcinoma. *Cancer Res.* 63:1454-1457.

31. Cohen,Y., Xing,M., Mambo,E., Guo,Z., Wu,G., Trink,B., Beller,U., Westra,W.H., Ladenson,P.W., and Sidransky,D. 2003. BRAF mutation in papillary thyroid carcinoma. *J. Natl. Cancer Inst.* 95:625-627.

32. Soares,P., Trovisco,V., Rocha,A.S., Lima,J., Castro,P., Preto,A., Maximo,V., Botelho,T., Seruca,R., and Sobrinho-Simoes,M. 2003. BRAF mutations and RET/PTC rearrangements are alternative events in the etiopathogenesis of PTC. *Oncogene* 22:4578-4580.

33. Nikiforova,M.N., Kimura,E.T., Gandhi,M., Biddinger,P.W., Knauf,J.A., Basolo,F., Zhu,Z., Giannini,R., Salvatore,G., Fusco,A. et al 2003. BRAF Mutations in Thyroid Tumors Are Restricted to Papillary Carcinomas and Anaplastic or Poorly Differentiated Carcinomas Arising from Papillary Carcinomas. *J Clin. Endocrinol. Metab* 88:5399-5404.

34. Xing,M., Westra,W.H., Tufano,R.P., Cohen,Y., Rosenbaum,E., Rhoden,K.J., Carson,K.A., Vasko,V., Larin,A., Tallini,G. et al 2005. BRAF mutation predicts a poorer clinical prognosis for papillary thyroid cancer. *J. Clin. Endocrinol. Metab.* 90:6373-6379.

35. Elisei,R., Ugolini,C., Viola,D., Lupi,C., Biagini,A., Giannini,R., Romei,C., Miccoli,P., Pinchera,A., and Basolo,F. 2008. BRAF(V600E) mutation and outcome of patients with papillary thyroid carcinoma: a 15-year median follow-up study. *J. Clin. Endocrinol. Metab.* 93:3943-3949.

36. Ricarte-Filho,J.C., Ryder,M., Chitale,D.A., Rivera,M., Heguy,A., Ladanyi,M., Janakiraman,M., Solit,D., Knauf,J.A., Tuttle,R.M. et al 2009. Mutational profile of advanced primary and metastatic radioactive iodine-refractory thyroid cancers reveals distinct pathogenetic roles for BRAF, PIK3CA, and AKT1. *Cancer Res.* 69:4885-4893.

37. Durante,C., Puxeddu,E., Ferretti,E., Morisi,R., Moretti,S., Bruno,R., Barbi,F., Avenia,N., Scipioni,A., Verrienti,A. et al 2007. BRAF mutations in papillary thyroid carcinomas inhibit genes involved in iodine metabolism. *J Clin Endocrinol Metab.* 92:2840-2843.

38. Ho,A.L., Grewal,R.K., Leboeuf,R., Sherman,E.J., Pfister,D.G., Deandreis,D., Pentlow,K.S., Zanzonico,P.B., Haque,S., Gavane,S. et al 2013. Selumetinib-enhanced radioiodine uptake in advanced thyroid cancer. *N. Engl. J. Med.* 368:623-632.

39. Kopetz,S., Desai,J., Chan,E., Hecht,J.R., O'dwyer,P.J., Lee,R.J., Nolop,K., and Saltz,L. 2010. PLX4032 in metastatic colorectal cancer patients with BRAF tumors. *J Clin Oncol* 28:7s (Abstr.)

40. Sturm,O.E., Orton,R., Grindlay,J., Birtwistle,M., Vyshemirsky,V., Gilbert,D., Calder,M., Pitt,A., Kholodenko,B., and Kolch,W. 2010. The mammalian MAPK/ERK pathway exhibits properties of a negative feedback amplifier. *Sci. Signal.* 3:ra90.

41. Montero-Conde,C., Ruiz-Llorente,S., Dominguez,J.M., Knauf,J.A., Viale,A., Sherman,E.J., Ryder,M., Ghossein,R.A., Rosen,N., and Fagin,J.A. 2013. Relief of Feedback Inhibition of HER3 Transcription by RAF and MEK Inhibitors Attenuates Their Antitumor Effects in BRAF-Mutant Thyroid Carcinomas. *Cancer Discov.* 3:520-533.

42. Prahallad,A., Sun,C., Huang,S., Di,N.F., Salazar,R., Zecchin,D., Beijersbergen,R.L., Bardelli,A., and Bernards,R. 2012. Unresponsiveness of colon cancer to BRAF(V600E) inhibition through feedback activation of EGFR. *Nature.*10.

43. Corcoran,R.B., Ebi,H., Turke,A.B., Coffee,E.M., Nishino,M., Cogdill,A.P., Brown,R.D., Pelle,P.D., Dias-Santagata,D., Hung,K.E. et al 2012. EGFR-mediated re-activation of MAPK signaling contributes to insensitivity of BRAF mutant colorectal cancers to RAF inhibition with vemurafenib. *Cancer Discov.* 2:227-235.

44. Flaherty,K.T., Infante,J.R., Daud,A., Gonzalez,R., Kefford,R.F., Sosman,J., Hamid,O., Schuchter,L., Cebon,J., Ibrahim,N. et al 2012. Combined BRAF and MEK inhibition in melanoma with BRAF V600 mutations. *N. Engl. J. Med.* 367:1694-1703.

45. Solit,D.B., and Rosen,N. 2014. Towards a unified model of RAF inhibitor resistance. *Cancer Discov.* 4:27-30.

46. Lawrence,M.S., Stojanov,P., Polak,P., Kryukov,G.V., Cibulskis,K., Sivachenko,A., Carter,S.L., Stewart,C., Mermel,C.H., Roberts,S.A. et al 2013. Mutational heterogeneity in cancer and the search for new cancer-associated genes. *Nature.* 499:214-218.

47. Rosove,M.H., Peddi,P.F., and Glaspy,J.A. 2013. BRAF V600E inhibition in anaplastic thyroid cancer. *N. Engl. J. Med.* 368:684-685.

48. Willyard,C. 2013. 'Basket studies' will hold intricate data for cancer drug approvals. *Nat. Med.* 19:655.

49. Lipson,E.J., and Drake,C.G. 2011. Ipilimumab: An Anti-CTLA-4 Antibody for Metastatic Melanoma. *Clinical Cancer Research* 17:6958-6962.

50. Freeman,G.J., Long,A.J., Iwai,Y., Bourque,K., Chernova,T., Nishimura,H., Fitz,L.J., Malenkovich,N., Okazaki,T., Byrne,M.C. et al 2000. Engagement of the Pd-1 Immunoinhibitory Receptor by a Novel B7 Family Member Leads to Negative Regulation of Lymphocyte Activation. *The Journal of Experimental Medicine* 192:1027-1034.

51. Cunha,L.L., Marcello,M.A., Morari,E.C., Nonogaki,S., Conte,F.F., Gerhard,R., Soares,F.A., Vassallo,J., and Ward,L.S. 2013. Differentiated thyroid carcinomas may elude the immune system by B7H1 upregulation. *Endocr. Relat Cancer.* 20:103-110.

52. Ryder,M., Callahan,M., Postow,M.A., Wolchok,J., and Fagin,J.A. 2014. Endocrine-related adverse events following ipilimumab in patients with advanced melanoma: a comprehensive retrospective review from a single institution. *Endocr. Relat Cancer.* 21:371-381.

53. Sadelain,M., Brentjens,R., and Riviere,I. 2013. The basic principles of chimeric antigen receptor design. *Cancer Discov.* 3:388-398.

www.ingramcontent.com/pod-product-compliance
Lightning Source LLC
Chambersburg PA
CBHW081842170526
45167CB00007B/2885